The Wellness Community Guide to
Fighting for Recovery from Cancer

THE WELLNESS COMMUNITY GUIDE TO FIGHTING FOR RECOVERY FROM CANCER

Harold H. Benjamin, Ph.D.

Revised and Expanded Edition of
From Victim to Victor

Jeremy P. Tarcher/Penguin
a member of
Penguin Group (USA) Inc.
New York

Please note: This book provides a unique source of information, guidance, inspiration, and hope for any patient who wants to take an active role in fighting cancer. The author believes in the methods designed to improve the quality of life of cancer patients and help them to become "Patients Active." However, this book should not replace your physician. The author expressly advises you to discuss the advice in this book with your physician. Responsibility for any adverse effects or unforeseen consequences from the use of the information contained in this book is expressly disclaimed by the publisher and the author.

Jeremy P. Tarcher/Penguin
a member of
Penguin Group (USA) Inc.
375 Hudson Street
New York, NY 10014
www.penguin.com

Library of Congress Cataloging in Publication Data

Benjamin, Harold H.
    The wellness community guide to fighting for recovery from cancer
/ Harold H. Benjamin ; foreword by Susan Love.—Rev. and expanded
ed. of From victim to victor.
        p.   cm.
    Originally published: Los Angeles : J.P. Tarcher, under title,
From victim to victor, 1987.
    Includes bibliographical references and index.
    ISBN 0-87477-794-1
    1. Cancer—Psychological aspects.   2. Cancer—Psychosomatic
aspects.   I. Title.
RC262.B36   1995   95-11417 CIP
362.1'96994—dc20

Design by Kate Nichols

Cover design by Susan Shankin

Printed in the United States of America

                16 17 18 19 20

This book is printed on acid-free paper.♾

CONTENTS

III   SPECIFIC METHODS TO FIGHT FOR RECOVERY

PROFESSIONAL ADVISORY BOARD

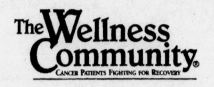

At this time, well over one thousand physicians throughout the United States refer their patients to Wellness Community facilities; there are over three hundred physicians serving on The Wellness Community's Professional Advisory Boards. Those serving on the Professional Advisory Board of The Wellness Community–National are:

Herbert Benson, M.D.
Chief, Section on Behavioral
　Medicine,
President, Mind/Body
　Medical Institute,
New England Deaconess
　Hospital

Armando E. Giuliano, M.D.
Director, Joyce Eisenberg
　Keefer Breast Center,
St. John's Hospital and Health
　Center

John Glick, M.D.
Director, University of
　Pennsylvania Cancer Center

Jimmie Holland, M.D.
Chief, Psychiatry Service,
Memorial Sloan-Kettering
　Cancer Center

Susan Love, M.D.
Director, Revlon/UCLA
　Breast Center,
University of California, Los
　Angeles

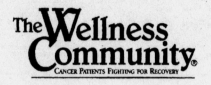

The Wellness Community®
CANCER PATIENTS FIGHTING FOR RECOVERY

FACULTY OF THE BEN B. & JOYCE C. EISENBERG
NATIONAL TRAINING CENTER

Mitch Golant, Ph.D., Clinical Psychologist, Chairperson

Lola Fisher, M.A., MFCC

Sang Eeta Levy, Ph.D., MFCC

Ruth Salk, M.A., MFCC

Malcolm Schultz, MFCC

Janet Smith, Ph.D., Clinical Psychologist

Lynne Weingarten, MFCC

Karen Wurtzel, M.S.W., LCSW

PROGRAM DIRECTOR OF
THE BEN B. & JOYCE C. EISENBERG
NATIONAL TRAINING CENTER

Michael Paige States, M.A., MFCC

Acknowledgments & Dedication

I acknowledge the importance of and dedicate this book to:

- The thousands of cancer patients who have permitted me to be a part of their lives and learn from them how important each day is and that every problem is not a major problem and there are many matters in life more important than "getting ahead"

- Lauren Benjamin, who has been my colleague and of valuable assistance in every aspect of this book

- The professional and administrative staff of The Wellness Community–National, whose every action is based on the ideal of integrity, selflessness, and generosity with only one thought in mind—being of as much help as possible to as many cancer patients as possible

- Joyce Eisenberg Keefer, whose generosity has made it possible for The Wellness Community to grow from psychosocially supporting 500 participants each week in 1984 to over 3,500 each week in 1995. Without her help, such growth would not have been possible.

FOREWORD

One of the major contributions to the psychosocial support of people with cancer in this country has come not from the medical profession but from an enthusiastic, dedicated layman who had a vision. Harold Benjamin started the Wellness Community after his wife was treated for breast cancer. Over the years the Wellness Community has grown to include thirteen facilities across the country, and it continues to thrive. It thrives in large part because it helps people with cancer focus on wellness rather than disease. Over the years Harold Benjamin has refined his vision, and now he presents it for us in this timely book, which will allow anyone to benefit from the philosophy of the Wellness Community and to become a "Patient Active."

There is one statement I hate making more than any other: "I am sorry, I have bad news for you. You have cancer." There is no way I can say these words and make them sound good. This is bad news to the recipient any way I phrase it. And there is one reaction—shock. Everyone I have known has reacted first with a feeling of total shock. *This can't be true. She isn't talking about me. It must be some mistake.* The shock is overwhelming, numbing and universal. Eventually it wears off, and that is when the differences among individuals become apparent. That is when they must each choose how to deal with this unwelcome visitor in their life. It is a choice, and an important one. It is this choice that Harold Benjamin and the Wellness Community address so comprehensively in this book. Does it matter? Well, as Harold Benjamin suggests, you will probably improve the quality of your life when you become a Patient Active. Is it possible you might even live longer? Everything is possible.

Although many of us have believed for a long time that there is a mind-body connection, the recent work of David Spiegel and his colleagues at Stanford University School of Medicine gave that connection scientific grounding. He studied women with metastatic breast cancer, some of whom participated in a support group in addition to receiving regular care, and others who did not. When he followed up on the women many years later he found to his surprise that those women who had participated in the support group had lived on average eighteen months longer than those who had not. This remarkable study proved once and for all that there is indeed a physical change that comes with support and community. The support group relied on many of the approaches advocated in this book: visualization, stress reduction, attention to doctor-patient and interpersonal relationships. Why do these ephemeral "touchy-feely" approaches to cancer recovery work? I am convinced that they change the environment of the cancer and help tip the balance against the cancer cell and in the patient's favor. Do they always work? Of course not. Nothing "always works." But they may well work for you. And what do you have to lose?

Harold Benjamin gives you his "almost promise" that you will feel better no matter what. So what are you waiting for? You have followed all of your doctor's prescriptions; now it is time to follow your own and become a Patient Active. You'll change the environment around you, you and your family will feel better, and—who knows—maybe the cancer will feel worse.

—Susan Love, M.D.
Director, Revlon/UCLA Breast Center

PREFACE

There is the often told biblical tale of the stranger who, many, many years ago, approaches the renowned cleric and makes the following offer: "If you can tell me the essence of your religion while standing on one leg, I will convert to your religion." Without hesitation the cleric responds, "Do not do unto others what thou wouldst not have done to thyself. This is the whole law. The rest is commentary."

The power of that statement is contained in its simplicity and the fact that it's all-encompassing and complete. The basic premise of this book, the Patient Active concept, and The Wellness Community can also be summarized in one similarly simple statement:

> Cancer patients who participate in their fight for recovery along with their physicians and health care professionals may enhance the possibility of their recovery and probably will improve the quality of their lives.

That says it all. The rest is commentary—explanations as to why that's true and how you, as a cancer patient, can take action that will probably result in your being happier and may enhance the possibility of your recovery—in short, becoming a Patient Active.

I

INTRODUCTION

CHAPTER 1

⌒∿

How to Fight for
Recovery from Cancer

If you have cancer, this guidebook is for you. I am writing it because, like your family, friends, physicians, and health care team, I want you to recover—above everything else, I want you to recover, and I will tell you why farther along in this chapter. You, I presume, are reading this book for the same reason you undergo chemotherapy, radiation, surgery, or immunotherapy— the hope for recovery. And since many of you are willing to fight for that recovery as partners with your physicians, this book will be your guide—your how-to book—how to fight for recovery from cancer.

As you will see, this book isn't about coping with cancer, learning to live with cancer, making the best of it, or dying from it. It's about fighting to recover, and if possible, recovering and enjoying life to the fullest while fighting. From it you will learn the psychological and emotional efforts you can use to fight for your recovery, why those efforts may alter the course of the illness toward health, and how, when, and where to use them to the greatest possible effect. And you will be joining the 30,000 cancer patients who have fought for recovery from cancer at The Wellness Community since we opened in 1982 and the 3,500 participants in thirteen cities who now participate in the program each week. On your team will also be the 350 physicians who serve on our Professional Advisory Boards and the more than 1,000 physicians who refer their patients to us.

One fact you should know at the very outset of our journey together is that the belief that everyone dies of cancer is a myth. There are millions of people in the United States to whom cancer is a memory. Not all cancer patients recover, but many of them do—many more than the myths would have you believe. The American Cancer Society's *Cancer Facts and Figures for 1995* reports that "over 8,000,000 Americans alive today have a history of cancer." Let that information sink in so that you know it at gut level—there are millions of people in the United States today to whom cancer is a memory. I know many of them and you will meet quite a few of them in this book. My wife, Harriet, is one of them.

Of course, there are no promises or guarantees of recovery or extended life either at The Wellness Community or in this book. Cancer is a serious illness. But there is hope and there is hard, scientific evidence which gives us reason to believe that there are actions you can take that may enhance your body's ability to fight for recovery. So, we have a fine line to walk. On one hand, you should know that there are actions you can take to join with your physician in the fight for recovery and that your participation *may* make recovery more likely. On the other hand, it must be absolutely clear that there is no inference or implication that if you enter the fight, things are certain to turn out as you want them to. As my mentor Norman Cousins said, "Biology sometimes overcomes psychology."

Another myth that must be shattered is that life ends with the diagnosis—that from that second on there is no longer any possibility of joy, fun, intimacy, work, and all other facets of life that make it worth living. That's just not true. I know hundreds and hundreds of people fighting to recover from cancer who are living full and complete lives within the confines of the illness. You can too. Your friends in this book will lead the way.

While there are no promises or guarantees in this book, there are two "almost" promises. First there is the promise that "almost" all cancer patients who become active in the fight for recovery will enjoy an improved quality of life—making the bad times less onerous and the good times even better. This almost promise is reinforced by a statement made by Robert Lowitz, M.D., Chief of Oncology at John Muir Medical Center, at a meeting of physicians discussing The Wellness Community. He said, "What I see as a provider, when the patients come back from their weekly visits or however often the two or three hundred patients a week go to The Wellness Community (where they use the Patient Active methods), is that the somatic symptoms of the patient are lessened. Their anxiety is lessened. Their depression is lessened and their energy level is up and they're psychologically and emotionally better." How about that!

The second almost promise is based upon the experience of many ex–cancer patients who tell us that the lessons learned fighting cancer improved their relationships and lives after cancer. Hopefully, that will happen to you. But remember, while these almost promises are important, they are peripheral to the main thrust of this book, your fight for recovery.

Now, since we will be going down this road together, there are a few other matters we should get clear between us. First, the psychological and social (psychosocial) methods suggested here are in support of and in addition to medical treatment. Not alternatives. Your physician and health care team are your first line of defense against the illness. If I had to choose be-tween medical treatment and psychosocial treatment, I would choose medical. Luckily, that is not a choice you have to make. You can use both. Thousands of Wellness Community partici-pants have.

Second, it is important for you to know that there is no way to follow any of these suggestions improperly or inadequately. What-ever you do, you are doing correctly and as well as it can be done. You should also know that if you try only some of the suggestions or ignore them completely, then that decision is the right decision for you. I truly believe that when deciding what actions you will take in your fight for recovery you can make no mistakes. In this area you are the perfect you. We have enough in life to feel guilty or inadequate about.

Another fact that requires great care in the telling is that our behavior and how we react to life events affects our health. Because of the way that message is sometimes delivered, it often leads cancer patients to believe that the messenger is implying that the patient is responsible for the onset of the illness or somehow at fault if the illness does not progress as hoped. Nothing could be farther from the truth. You are not, and cannot be, responsible for the illness, and it is not, and cannot be, your fault if the disease is not progressing as hoped. We will discuss this issue more thoroughly in Chapters 31 and 32. Again, this is a fine line we must walk—gathering inspiration and hope while not blaming yourself if things are not going as you want them to. I'm sure we can walk that fine line together.

Third, I am not suggesting that changes in behavior are easy or uncomplicated. They are not. They take effort and determination. However, the only side effects of attempting to make those changes is a better quality of life. Think about that—the only side effect of fighting for recovery is becoming happier.

Fourth, the basic premise of this book—that there are actions you can take which may have a positive effect on the course of the illness—is no pie-in-the-sky claim or one to be taken lightly. It is supported by studies in the relatively new field called psychoneuroimmunology—PNI for short—popularly known as "the mind/body connection." Broadly speaking, PNI is the study of the effect emotions and mental activity have on physical well-being. In the opening chapter of the authoritative book *Mind/Body Medicine,* published in 1993, the editors state forthrightly that it has been scientifically established that the patient's actions can have a positive effect on the course of an illness:

> For patients [knowing that the mind effects the body] has a practical significance. It means that by paying attention to and exerting some control over emotional and mental states you [the patient] may recover more rapidly from being sick and may be able to shorten the [course of illness] . . .

How about that!

As recently as thirty years ago that statement could not have been made. Patients had no options. When we were ill we were relegated to being passive spectators. Our physicians were active. It was they who were fighting for our recovery. Our role was limited and well defined. It included only complying with our physicians' instructions, accepting their ministrations, and if we were so inclined, praying for divine intervention. That was it. But that's no longer true. Now we know that you, as a cancer patient, can be a partner with your physician and that your participation may have a positive effect on the course of the illness. Here's the encouraging part—being and becoming an active participant in the fight for recovery is a skill that can be learned. You can do that right here— right now. In The Wellness Community, we call a person who has joined with his or her physician in the fight for recovery—who has become an active participant in that fight—a Patient Active. We consider that a title of distinction.

Fifth, it's never too late to start the fight for recovery. There are two reasons for that statement. The first is that whatever the stage of the illness when you start, you will probably improve the quality of your life. The second reason is that no matter when you start, there is the possibility that your actions may have a positive effect on the course of the illness. In his book *The Body Is the Hero,* Ronald Glasser, Ph.D., tells a dramatic story that illustrates why it's never too late to try.

A kidney containing undetected cancer cells was transplanted into a recipient who had received drugs to suppress his immune system. (Unless the immune system is suppressed by drugs, it will reject the transplanted organ.) Within days, the patient showed signs of cancer not only in his new kidney but also in his lungs. His doctors immediately deduced that the cancer had been introduced into his body by the transplanted kidney and had spread rapidly because his immune system had been rendered impotent by drugs. They discontinued the immune-suppressing drugs, and the cancer disappeared.

This story is a remarkable illustration of the power of the immune system. Weakened sufficiently by the drugs to permit cancer cells to grow and take hold, it was able, when it regained its strength, to kill the cancer cells that had already started to form a tumor.

Therefore, it's reasonable for you to hope that your immune system can be bolstered to reverse the course of the illness. No matter what the stage of the illness, every story of a recovered cancer patient teaches that same lesson.

WHY THE WELLNESS COMMUNITY GUIDEBOOK?

Before answering that question, a brief history is in order. The Wellness Community resulted from my study of the field of the psychological treatment of cancer patients which began when my wife, Harriet, had both breasts removed because of cancer in 1972. She is fine today. After some nine years of study, in 1981, I conceived of the Patient Active concept, which I will describe as we go along, and one year later opened The Wellness Community in Santa Monica, California, based on that concept. I have been the full-time leader of the program, with one title or another, since we opened. Before that, I was a Beverly Hills attorney and businessman. When asked by members of the media and my friends why I retired as a lawyer to devote all my efforts to this program without pay, I am hard put to come up with an answer. The one thing I do know is that after Harriet's illness, for some reason, it was very important to me that as many people as possible recover from cancer to the greatest extent possible, and I thought I could help. And although I can't explain why, I was anxious to devote all my efforts to that undertaking, and I have done just that.

I have named this book for The Wellness Community because, in addition to the most current scientific information, it incorporates the techniques and methods developed and used there. Information about the services is described in Appendix 1. It also incorporates the advice and wisdom of hundreds and hundreds of cancer patients and ex–cancer patients, most of whom were Wellness Community participants.

You cannot imagine how much these Wellness Community participants and ex-participants want to help—how eager they are to pass on to you what they learned. They want you to know about fighting for recovery, living life to the fullest while fighting, overcoming the psychological and social problems brought about by cancer, the reasonableness and benefits of hope, the possibility that you can play an important part in the fight for recovery, and how your participation in that fight may, just may, achieve the result we all want—freedom from illness.

The Wellness Community is the program Gilda Radner wrote about in her book *It's Always Something*. Gilda described The Wellness Community in the following words:

I stopped sitting at home saying "Why me?" or being depressed thinking I was the only one. I began to crawl to The Wellness Community like someone in search of an oasis in the desert. My car couldn't get me there fast enough. I couldn't walk fast enough from the parking lot. I couldn't get inside fast enough to be nourished by other cancer patients, and to know that I was not alone. I could hire people to be around me, I could pay groups of people to go through this with me, but I could never get what I got there, not ever.

Much of what Gilda received at The Wellness Community in Santa Monica you can get from reading this book—you don't need a Wellness Community to become a Patient Active. You can do it by yourself with this book as your guide. I know that, because a great many cancer patients who have read *From Victim to Victor*, the first book to describe the Patient Active concept, published in 1988, told me that that's what they did.

You might find it interesting to know that at The Wellness Community we have seen so many people recover that we set up a special group for them. We call that group the Wellness Community Connection, because these recovered cancer patients want to stay connected with The Wellness Community to help others facing the problems they faced. But one word of caution here: Would those people who have recovered after becoming Patients Active have had the same result if they had never heard of The Wellness Community or joined with their physicians in their fight for recovery? Maybe. Maybe not. But no matter—we are happy that their illness turned out as it did, happy that we know them so that we can share in their joy, happy that they are a shining example of a key lesson to be learned: that many, many people recover from cancer and that it is always reasonable to have hope.

HOW TO USE THIS BOOK

This format does not require that you read the chapters in sequence. You can go immediately to the chapters that are most important to you. Part I (Chapters 1 through 4) focuses on knowledge about cancer and your fight for recovery generally. Most readers will find this section helpful in understanding the basis for the suggestions made in Part III. Part II (Chapters 5 through 10) discusses the effect of stress and methods of dealing with it—an important part of the fight for recovery. Part III (Chapters 11 through 36) sets forth the specific suggestions you can use, and Part IV (Questions 1 through 6) answers several pragmatic questions faced by cancer patients who decide to become Patients Active.

Also, I have arranged to introduce you to many ex–cancer patients throughout this book, because I know that a most important part of the fight for recovery is maintaining hope in the face of the distress brought about by cancer, and that meeting or learning about ex–cancer patients always restores hope. So meet them you will. Those ex-patients are the real experts on how to fight for recovery, and I want to be the direct connection between you and them so that you can use the methods they used and benefit from their experience.

Finally, in this book, I will not consider the physical or spiritual

aspects of cancer treatment—only the mental. Certainly, the physical, spiritual, and mental aspects of life cannot be completely
separated. All three are integral and important parts of total cancer
patient care. But since medical matters are best left in the competent hands of the medical profession and spiritual matters are best
left to the clergy, this book will concern itself only with the area in
which The Wellness Community is an acknowledged leader—the
effect that the psychological, emotional, social, and philosophical
aspects of our lives have on the possibility of recovery.

Now, let's get on with the specifics. The first message of hope
from an ex–cancer patient is from a woman I know reasonably
well—Harriet Benjamin. Here is her answer to the question "Do
you believe that the cancer patient can play a part in his or her fight
for recovery?"

*I truly believe there is much cancer patients can do which may help them
recover. I was diagnosed with breast cancer in 1972. I was sure I was going
to die. It all came about so quickly. I had quite a bit of cancer in my family,
and it was common knowledge that everyone who had cancer died of it.
Before I knew it, I was on the table and the biopsy was done and the
modified radical mastectomy was complete—all at one session. Because at
that time Harold and I were involved in a social movement in Santa
Monica based upon self-reliance, I knew that it was important that I fight
for my recovery and not be passive in the face of adversity, and I did just
that. I did everything I could think of to be partners with my medical team.
Less than a year later, I had the second mastectomy. They didn't have
lumpectomies in those days. I continued the fight to recover. I believe that
my physicians and medical team were superb. I also believe that my fight
played a large part in bringing about the fact that it is more than twenty
years later and I have neither breasts nor symptoms. The common knowledge that everyone dies of cancer was wrong. Hooray!*

Harriet Benjamin

CHAPTER 2

~2~

You Have Power to Fight
for Your Recovery

The proof that you are not helpless in your fight for recovery starts with an analogy. You are driving down the highway and suddenly your car just stops. If you are as mechanically unskilled as I am, you are helpless. You have no alternative but to push the car to the side of the road, call a mechanic, and then stand by and watch the mechanic while all the other cars go whizzing by. Sadly, many cancer patients deal with their bodies the way they deal with their cars—by turning them over to someone who can "fix" bodies, usually called "doctor," and doing nothing but watching and hoping that the doctor will succeed.

But the human body is not like an automobile which can't fix itself. When illness or injury occurs, except in the most extreme cases, our bodies automatically—without conscious effort on our part—do everything necessary to return to normalcy without help from any outside source. Physicians call that effort to maintain normalcy homeostasis.

Cancer is one of those extreme cases where the body needs help. But that doesn't mean that the body is helpless—that all of its ability to fight for recovery has been dissipated. It still has quite a bit of that recuperative power and is fighting for recovery whether you know it or not. Think of a man who falls into a hole too deep to climb out. When help appears and a rope is thrown down, the man uses his strength to climb out of the hole. Just because he is in a difficult situation doesn't mean he is powerless. He had plenty of power, just not enough to get out of the hole himself. In the same manner, your body probably still has plenty of power, just not enough to fight this disease without help.

But there is a matter of concern here. We are learning that there is the possibility that your body may not be fighting to its full capacity—not using all of its powers—because of the way you are reacting to life events. And since the harder your body works to fight off the illness the more likely your recovery, that unhealthy way of reacting to life events should and can be corrected.

To understand the methodology for correcting that condition, you should be aware of the following hypothesis emanating from the study of the connection between the mind and the body: The immune system, the body's first line of defense against cancer, is relatively lethargic in the body of a cancer patient who feels hopeless, helpless, and passive, while that same system will be more active and energetic in the body of a person who has hope and a fighting spirit. It therefore behooves cancer patients to be hopeful and determined to recover. And this book is designed to help you, as a cancer patient, do just that.

THE PATIENT ACTIVE CONCEPT

As a further clarification of the methodology and as the beginning of the discussion of the Patient Active concept, assume a scale of 1 to 10 with 10 representing the pinnacle of hope and fighting spirit—the point at which your immune system will fight most vigorously and energetically. Let's assume further that, at the time of reading this book, you are a 6. The methods suggested here are designed so that by their use your hope and fighting spirit will be enhanced to a 10 and your recuperative powers will be working as hard as they can. By taking affirmative, conscious action to fight for recovery, you will join the two partners already engaged in that battle—your body, automatically fighting for recovery, and your physician. You are using the Patient Active concept. You have become a Patient Active.

Definition: The Patient Active concept is a unique and revolutionary method which combines two disciplines—psychology and psychoneuroimmunology (PNI). The study of PNI has revealed and documented that emotions and mental activity affect the functions of the body—both positively and negatively. The Patient Active concept seeks to apply psychological methods to stimulate the internal functions so that they will work to their full capacity to promote recovery. Some specific statements about the concept will be helpful:

- The Patient Active concept combines the will of the patient with the skill of the physician. A powerful combination.
- The Patient Active concept is a series of psychological and emotional guidelines cancer patients can use which may enhance the possibility of recovery.
- The Patient Active concept is not designed to help cancer patients learn to die from or adapt their lives to cancer. It is designed to help cancer patients fight for their recovery along with their physicians and other health care professionals, in the expectation that such activity will probably improve the quality of their lives and the hope that it will enhance the possibility of their recovery.

WHO ARE PATIENTS ACTIVE?

Patients Active are those cancer patients who believe that they are not helpless in the face of cancer, that there are actions they can take to fight for recovery which will improve the quality of their lives and may enhance the possibility of their recovery, and who exert the effort necessary to learn what those actions are and to put some of them into practice as partners with their physicians.

Choosing to be a Patient Active is not a single monumental choice; it is a series of small decisions to fight for recovery, rather than turn all of the responsibility over to the physician.

Most cancer patients, when they first hear the diagnosis, are despondent, frightened, certain they have no chance of recovery, and convinced they are helpless. Perhaps you recognize those feelings. But often many of those feelings change when they become Patients Active. Yes, they are concerned and anxious, frightened and apprehensive. But they are fighting, and not fighting alone. They know that there is hope and that they are not helpless. They act optimistic and, to the best of their ability, energetic, and because of all that, life becomes more livable, more pleasant. And all of that is available to you. I know it is. I have seen it happen to hundreds of cancer patients just like you.

I was a fifty-seven-year-old real estate developer in 1984 when I was diagnosed with late-stage lymphoma, cancer of the lymphatic system, and my doctor told me my chances of recovery were slim. I remember I spent the days immediately after receiving the diagnosis talking about suicide. I would often burst into tears. I had given up and I was sure I was going to die soon. Although I had a family and friends, I felt alone. I wouldn't let them be with me. They couldn't understand—they didn't have cancer; they weren't doomed to die.

But Marsha, my wife, urged me to try The Wellness Community. Although I was depressed and could hardly walk, and was still sure I was going to die, I went. I met all those people who were fighting for recovery and didn't seem nearly as depressed as I was. I joined a group, started to do directed visualization, changed my diet, began to learn about cancer, took back control of many areas of my life, and started to act like a human being again, and wonderful things started to happen. The crying spells vanished, I started to enjoy life for the first time in many months, and my physical condition started to improve. Today, almost twelve years later, I am still without symptoms. Up until two years ago I was back at work full-time. Now, I'm retired, but still taking good care of myself. I am absolutely convinced that my participation in my fight for recovery played an invaluable role in my recovery. I don't believe I would have survived if I had not had wonderful medical treatment, and if I had not taken the actions I did to help myself get well. Without either I was a goner.

                                                              Phil

CHAPTER 3

Why These Methods Help

I believe that the methods of fighting for recovery suggested here will be more meaningful and easily accomplished if there is an understanding of the "surveillance theory," subscribed to by most physicians, which undergirds each of those suggestions. For that reason, I have reduced the concept to its bare essentials. A more thorough examination of the theory may be found in Part IV, Questions 3 and 4.

THE ESSENTIALS OF THE THEORY

1. We all have cancer cells proliferating in our bodies much of the time.
2. One of the functions of the immune system is to destroy cancer cells as they appear. In the majority of cases, the immune system gets rid of the cancer cells before they can do any harm.
3. Cancer results when the immune system is not strong enough to destroy the cancer cells as they appear. If the immune system does not rid the body of them relatively quickly they will "take hold" and cause the problems we are all familiar with.
4. Thus, since you have cancer, it appears that cancer cells appeared in your body and your immune system was not strong enough to destroy them.

5. It is believed by many scientists that when cancer has already taken hold, if the immune system becomes stronger it may become strong enough to destroy the cancer cells already there and make recovery more likely.

6. For that reason—to strengthen the immune system—for some cancers and under certain circumstances, physicians administer chemicals such as interleukin-2 and interferon.

7. The immune system is strengthened by pleasant emotions and suppressed by long-term, unremitting unpleasant emotions, often called stress.

8. Therefore, for the same reason that interleukin-2 and interferon are prescribed for cancer patients—to strengthen the immune system in the hope that it will become strong enough to have a positive effect on the course of the illness—every method suggested here is designed to maximize pleasant emotions (improve the quality of life) and minimize unpleasant emotions (stress).

Because of the importance of items 7 and 8 above, I will reiterate them in a slightly different form as follows:

• There is a reasonable possibility that if your immune system becomes stronger it may alter the course of the illness toward health.

• Long-term, unremitting unpleasant emotions depress and pleasant emotions enhance the immune system.

• Therefore, all the methods suggested here are designed to attempt to limit the number, duration, and intensity of unpleasant emotions and maximize the number, duration, and intensity of pleasant emotions.

CHAPTER 4

∾

The "Almost" Promise

There are very few promises or guarantees to be made in the area of fighting cancer, but I now make a statement I believe you can rely on: *If you become a Patient Active, you probably will improve the quality of your life.* Notice, I did not use the words "may" or "might." I said "probably"—a much more positive word. And this is not just a Wellness Community notion. J. C. Holland, M.D., Chief of Psychiatry at Memorial Sloan-Kettering Cancer Center, an authority on the psychological and emotional aspects of cancer, had the following to say, without equivocation, in her chapter in *Mind/Body Medicine:* ". . . mind/body approaches including support groups; counseling; and control of anxiety, depression and pain—can have a tremendous impact on the cancer patient's quality of life."

How about that? Mind/body approaches can have a "tremendous impact on the cancer patient's quality of life." There's the "almost" promise: If you become a Patient Active—if you use some or all of the techniques you can learn here—you may not only enhance the possibility of your recovery, as described in the previous chapter, but, as an added bonus, you will probably improve the quality of your life. A significant benefit under any circumstances.

Once again, science is not the only source of this exciting information. I have also learned about the happiness-improving qualities of being a Patient Active from thousands of cancer patients

and ex--cancer patients. Many have attributed to their cancer experience better relationships with their family and friends, a newfound ability to stop and smell the roses, an enhanced love for those
around them, an openness that they never had before, the ability to
ask for what they want, and generally, a much improved quality of
life. Perhaps the most important part of the life changes brought
about by becoming active in the fight for recovery is their realization of just how much control they have over their lives. See if that's
happening for you. If it's not, that doesn't mean that you are doing
something wrong. All it means is that your circumstances are different. Perhaps you might want to take some affirmative action, like
Lilly, a nurse I met at a lecture I gave in 1990.

Lilly wrote to me about a year after we met and told me that
she had had a mastectomy in 1989 and had read my book but did
nothing about it, believing the effort wasn't worth it. All she did
was follow her doctor's instructions and nothing more; she was
miserable and her health continued to deteriorate. Soon after the
lecture, her three-year-old daughter become quite ill, and when
she thought the little girl was going to die Lilly learned how
precious life was and how her passivity had cheated her and her
daughter out of a great deal of joy.

> Because I wanted to watch my little girl grow up and I
> believed that by my actions I might have an effect on the illness
> and that, in any event, I could enjoy life while going through
> this ordeal, I took control of my life. I left a department in the
> hospital I hated and went to the nursery. I had several long
> talks with my husband and mother, telling them what I
> wanted from our relationship, I practiced the Relaxation Re-
> sponse and it all worked—I'm happy for the first time in over
> three years and I'm a good mother to my daughter, and my
> relationships with my husband and mother are better than they
> were before I was ill. I'm not well yet and there are still things I
> can't do the way I did before, but I'm better than I was. I don't
> know for sure whether my newfound power has anything to
> do with that, but I'd be surprised if it didn't.

Cancer changes many of the day-to-day aspects of living, but the pursuit of happiness can go on during the fight for recovery if you want it to and make the necessary changes. Many cancer patients not only pursue happiness while fighting for recovery but find their enjoyment of life heightened because cancer has taught them what a precious gift life is.

At The Wellness Community we see hundreds of people who, while fighting cancer, are raising children, operating businesses, holding down jobs, practicing medicine, falling in or out of love. We see others whose activities are to some extent restricted by the illness but who continue to laugh, read, plan for the future, help other cancer patients, and do many of the things they did before the illness, within their current abilities. On the other hand, if you expect life to be miserable, it will probably be just that. Of course, whether or not life is worth living is a matter of individual and personal perception. To one person, life with pain may be well worth fighting for. For another, the inability to do all that she did before the illness may make life intolerable.

As you are reading this, do not interpret the message to be: "Don't be depressed," or, "Stop crying and get on with your life." These phrases are unrealistic, either as an admonition or as well-intentioned advice. Cancer is bad news. It's something to be worried about. However, the point here is that there can be a good quality of life with and after cancer—life worth living, for those who want it, expect it, work for it, and whose circumstances permit it.

Of course, being happy is dependent, to a great extent, on how you feel physically. It's difficult, and sometimes impossible, to feel joy when you are in pain or nauseated. But for most cancer patients, those periods come and go. They are usually not permanent. This off-and-on phenomenon was described by Louise, who was battling a long-standing melanoma, and is still under treatment as of the writing of this book. Speaking to a group of cancer patients new to The Wellness Community, Louise said:

Because I was faced with the battle of and for my life I was forced to pay attention to how precious every day and every moment was. Life with cancer is tough. When the treatments or the cancer make you feel lousy or you receive bad news, life doesn't seem like a bowl of cherries, and if you are left without a clue as to what to do and feeling helpless, life is even tougher. I know. I am there right now. But there are many periods of my life when I don't feel all that bad, and during those times, I use my Patient Active tools and become a fighter, and I fight not only for life but for happiness—and that fight I often win. Life doesn't become a bowl of cherries, but it becomes a lot better.

She ended with the encouraging phrase "It can happen for you." And perhaps it already has. Perhaps it's still to come. Too bad that we need the trauma of cancer to alert us to what life is all about.

11

Control Stress
to Fight
for Recovery

CHAPTER 5

The Importance of
Controlling Stress—
Unpleasant Emotions—
as Part of Your Fight
for Recovery

NOTE: Before we go forward here, it will be helpful to notice that
the words "unpleasant emotions", "stress," and "distress" are used
interchangeably, as are the words "pleasant emotions" and "eustress". It is also important to know that although the suggested
actions do not ensure the results we want, I know of no instance,
either anecdotal or otherwise, that has suggested that the patient's
participation in the fight for recovery has had anything but a
beneficial effect. So you have everything to gain and nothing
to lose.

DISCUSSION: As you will remember from Chapter 3 and Part
IV, Questions 3 and 4, if you have read them yet, long-term
unremitting, unpleasant emotions—stress—depress the immune
system, and eustress—pleasant emotions—enhance the power of
the immune system—the body's first line of defense against cancer. Therefore, throughout this book, I am suggesting that as a part
of the fight for recovery, you attempt to maximize the intensity
and duration of eustress and minimize the intensity and duration of
stress.

The procedures for augmenting eustress are described in almost every chapter in this book, and particularly in Chapter 10.

The procedures for controlling particular unpleasant emotions are set forth in Chapters 11 through 36. However, the next four chapters are highlighted because they describe methods of dealing with and counteracting any and all unpleasant emotions—stress—without reference to a particular type of situation or emotion. To that extent, they are universal. When the specific methods aren't applicable, these methods can be relied on.

In order to use these general methods as effectively as possible, it will be important to know (1) what stress is, (2) where it comes from, and (3) what effect it has on our bodies.

Stress and its physical consequences always come about as follows:

STRESSOR ⟶	STRESS ⟶	PHYSICAL REACTION
EVENT	MENTAL REACTION	
An (1) event that (2) is perceived and (3) stimulates a mental reaction	The automatic mental reaction to the perception of a stressor	The automatic physical reaction that always follows the mental reaction to stress

An example of a stressor followed by stress is as follows: If you are walking down the street and observe a car passing, that event is not a stressor, since it does not evoke a mental reaction. However, if you see a long-lost friend in the car, that stressor evokes eustress—a happy reaction. Conversely, suppose you see a man in the car pointing a gun at you. Your automatic reaction is fear. The man in the car is the stressor. The fear is the stress. The physical reaction to stress is depression of the immune system.

The examples used are illustrations of short-term stress which, under all but the most unusual circumstances, have no lasting effects. It is the long-term stressors such as family, financial, marital, business difficulties, or unconscious stressors which depress the immune system. For that reason, if you experience such a long-term, unplesant stressor, it is in your best interest to take action to see to it that it continues for the shortest period of time, and that its intensity is at the lowest level, so it will have the least effect on the immune system. When an event evokes a pleasant emotion, it seems reasonable to do what is necessary to prolong and deepen the event and the emotion so as to strengthen your immune system.

I will digress here for just a moment to observe that the above advice is so simple and basic as to make it almost embarrassing to give it. Who, sick or well, would not want to minimize unpleasant emotions and maximize pleasant emotions? Yet I know, from talking to any number of cancer patients, that the very first time they gave any thought to a *conscious* effort to prolong happiness or shorten unhappiness was after they were diagnosed and became a part of The Wellness Community. Many recovered cancer patients report that they have learned this technique from their bout with cancer, and that it has changed their lives after cancer.

Of course, the emotion aroused by the stressor is dependent on the person who perceives the event. The same stressor may trigger a completely different reaction in two people perceiving the same event. Daughter Jill is dating John. Jill's father dislikes John. Her mother likes him. When Jill tells her parents that she and John have broken up, Father is happy and Mother is sad.

And it's not even necessary that the stressor take place in the world around you. It may take place only in your mind and concern matters of the past and future as well as the present. If you remember how much fun you had during the last holiday season, a pleasant emotion is aroused. If you anticipate an unpleasant task you soon must do, a disagreeable emotion is triggered. As you see, stress may be either distress or eustress. Let's discuss distress first.

CONTROL OF DISTRESS

Stress can be controlled in several ways, all of which will be discussed in Chapters 7, 8, 9, and 10. However, to be able to use any of the suggested methods, it will be necessary to first identify and acknowledge the unpleasant emotions. The method for doing that is discussed in the next chapter.

CHAPTER 6

Do Something About the Stressors in Your Life

We start by acknowledging that there are any number of stressors in life that are out of our control. You can't quit your job if you need the money or the insurance it provides. It's not easy to divorce a spouse, and there is really nothing we can do about the man in the car with the gun or the earthquake that rattles our world. For those unalterable stressors we can look to the Serenity Prayer which asks that the universe grant us the grace "to accept with serenity the things that cannot be changed, courage to change the things which should be changed, and the wisdom to know the difference."

However, there are many stressors over which you do have some control—which you can change. I know any number of people who have altered life circumstances when they believed that those circumstances were stressors suppressing their immune systems and perhaps hindering their fight for recovery, or when they realized that life was finite and it was madness to live under unhappy circumstances if they didn't have to. Some have gone so far as to quit jobs, leave spouses, return to spouses, move out of town, change doctors, become more assertive, become less assertive. Most changes, of course, are not as drastic and come about gradually. *The suggestion here is do whatever you can to become aware of your emotions as they cascade through your life, and then do something about them—do what you can to minimize the unpleasant emotions and maximize the pleasant emotions.* That's the general rule. The specifics are discussed throughout this book.

HOW TO RECOGNIZE EMOTIONS

In order to take action to control stress, you must first recognize and acknowledge it. You may be surprised that this type of analysis is necessary, but just like an illness, an emotion is difficult to "treat" unless it is diagnosed.

If you think about it, you will realize that when we experience an emotion, that's all we do—experience it. We may revel in a pleasant emotion and complain about an unpleasant emotion, but we don't consider the possibility that we might be able to augment the pleasant or diminish the unpleasant emotion. The suggestions made in this chapter are methods you can use to acknowledge—"diagnose"—an emotion so that you can take action to control it.

To fully benefit from the suggested processes for diagnosing an emotion, an understanding of the left brain / right brain theory will be helpful. Although recent research has suggested that the delineation between the activities of the right and left brain are not as clear and precise as once thought, it remains the perfect metaphor for a discussion of the methods I am suggesting.

The right brain / left brain theory posits that the left hemisphere of the brain, sometimes called the major hemisphere, governs problem solving and is pragmatic, businesslike, logical, materialistic, and mechanistic, while the right hemisphere is said to govern those aspects of our personalities which are emotional, ethereal, imaginative, romantic, artistic, sensual, and creative.

To illustrate the difference between right brain and left brain activity, compare a math problem with an emotion. When confronted with a math problem we immediately isolate and concentrate on the problem, attempt to understand it, consider it from all angles, use the knowledge available, and try to solve it. That's all done in the left hemisphere. Emotions, on the other hand, are experienced in the right hemisphere and are felt rather than understood. They may be, and often are, pervasive, but since, unless specific action is taken, they are never isolated and analyzed, they remain amorphous and blurry. In that form, it is almost impossible to deal with them. It's like seeing a forest whose beauty you can enjoy in the abstract, but if you want to use the lumber it produces, you must concentrate on one tree at a time.

By all of this I am suggesting that in order to use the methods suggested to control stress, you must first move the unpleasant emotion to the left side of the brain. Not an easy task. Very few of us have any practice at it. But I know it can be done. I've done it. I now recognize most of my emotions as they flit through my life.

I pause here to describe a personal experience that has been helpful to me, in the hope that you may find it useful. Many years ago—for reasons unknown to me and without any conscious effort—about every twenty minutes, my mind automatically went to the question "How are you feeling emotionally?" Of course, that was an internal appraisal. No one but me knew it was going on.

Most of the time the response to the question was neutral. But every so often, the answer came back: "You feel sad—unhappy—envious—insignificant—unworthy—ineffective." When that happened, I immediately sought to determine what caused the feeling, and quite often I was successful; quite often the reasons were childish, and with that realization, they disappeared. However, there were times when I realized that there were valid reasons for my reaction, and I attempted to take action to avoid the situation in the future and minimize the immediate reaction.

Sometimes the emotion that came up was pleasant, and I was equally unaware of its cause until I searched for it. Very often the cause was also childish. But who cared? I wanted more of that and took action to get it. Over the years, the clock has speeded up. I am now constantly, subconsciously and internally, asking myself the "How are you feeling emotionally?" question. I believe that drill, which moved the emotion to the left side of my brain, where it can be examined, makes my life happier.

That method is available to you. All it takes is determination to watch your emotions. You can also ask your friends to help you.

An example of that is an excerpt from a letter I received from Charles, a member of an audience of cancer patients, in response to my suggestion that they look for and change the stressors in their lives. I don't know what type of cancer Charles had. "Dear Dr. Benjamin," it began.

> I discussed your lecture with my brother David and asked him if he knew of any stressors I had. I couldn't think of any. Within the blink of an eye, he described several. One of them struck me as particularly strange that I had not seen it. David and I operate a small bookstore and we have one customer who buys a great many books from us. However, he always leaves books strewn around the store, when he comes in to browse. I didn't realize it, but David says that after that customer leaves, I am a different person for the rest of the day. And, as I thought about it, I saw he was right. I started to watch for the feeling, and when I found it, decided whether it was appropriate or not. That taught me how to watch for other emotional reactions to events that take place in my life, and when I find them, I think about them and decide whether they are appropriate or not. Sometimes they are—sometimes they're not. When they're not, I do my best to get rid of them. It has become like a game for me.

Stress—the unpleasant feeling—that comes about as a result of an incident, such as Charles described, is relatively easy to become aware of. You can watch for the incident—as Charles did—and see what your reaction is. You know why you become annoyed when someone does something obviously wrong.

The tricky stressors are those that arouse unpleasant feelings for no apparent reason. No one did anything obviously wrong or annoying and yet you still feel unhappy—depressed, demeaned—valueless. My experience is that if you watch for the feeling and, when you notice that you have it, if you attempt to determine what triggered it, you may learn that the unpleasant feeling is childish and not a reasonable adult reaction—in which case it will go away. If you can't find the reasons for them, you might discuss the matter with family or friends or clergy or perhaps a psychotherapist.

KEEP A "QUALITY OF LIFE" CHART

Another method for becoming aware of your emotions and moving them to the left side of your brain is the Quality of Life chart I have devised as indicated on page 34. Using these charts forces you to recognize, acknowledge, and name the emotion. Here's how that happens: First, you school yourself to be watchful of the emotions you are feeling. When you recognize one, such as anger, fear, anxiety, or envy, you name a chart in its honor. Or you can name the chart in the form of a question—How Happy Am I? How Healthy Am I? How Much Pain Am I In? How Is My Nausea? How Is My Social Life? How Is My Relationship with Dr. X? *By naming the chart you have recognized and acknowledged the emotion.* You have moved it to the left side of your brain. Every time you use that chart you will acknowledge the emotion.

You then assign a number to that emotion indicating its intensity: "I gave it a 5 yesterday—is that more or less than I feel today?" You have now created a problem to be solved which ensures that it will stay on the left side of your brain where you can deal with it.

CHART INSTRUCTIONS

- Become aware of the emotion.
- Make a chart with the name of the emotion.
- When you start the chart, put the date you start at the lower left-hand corner and place a dot at the number you believe identifies the intensity of that emotion at that moment. You have now transferred the emotion to the left side of the

brain, recognized, and acknowledged it. Now you can decide what, if anything, you should do about it.

- Make entries in the chart as often or as seldom as you like.
- When you make the next entry, place the date of that entry at the bottom of the chart on the first vertical line to the right of the starting line and place a dot at the numbered horizontal line that you believe symbolizes the way you feel then. Once again, the emotion is in a position to be considered. This happens every time you use the charts.

As you see, this method can be used for pleasant as well as unpleasant emotions. Pleasant emotions should also be analyzed, so as to get as much enjoyment as possible from them.

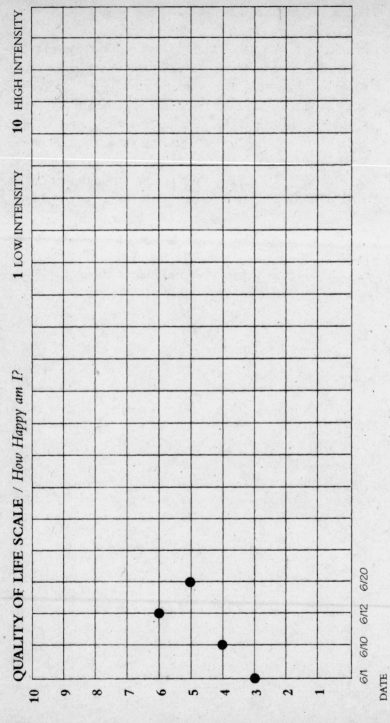

QUALITY OF LIFE SCALE / *How Happy am I?*

1 LOW INTENSITY   10 HIGH INTENSITY

34

CHAPTER 7

᠆

How to Re-form a Negative Emotion

As a prelude to this chapter, I believe we will agree that it's not possible or even desirable to change every negative emotion into a positive one. Sometimes it's appropriate to feel disagreeable emotions such as fear, guilt, or anxiety. Cancer is something to be fearful of. It's appropriate to feel guilty if you purposely hurt someone's feelings. It's reasonable to feel anxious if you believe you are about to lose your job. It's also reasonable to feel the hurt of a lost love or anxiety about one or another aspect of the future.

However, there are many circumstances when it is not so clear that your reaction is reasonable, and there is always the question of how long even a reasonable unpleasant emotion should be allowed to hang on. So, as part of your fight for recovery—to reduce the pressure on your immune system—the intensity of an emotion should be minimized. To do that you might ask yourself questions such as: Is the reaction reasonable? Has it continued for more than a reasonable period of time? The methods of dealing with unrealistic reactions and unpleasant emotions that have remained for too long are the subject of this chapter, with the complete understanding that you have the overriding concern of cancer, which must always be taken into account.

The case of Lynn, an entrepreneur whose partner had, she said, forced her out of the business she had started, is illustrative of an emotion that was intense and long-lasting and may have had an effect on the course of the illness. When Lynn's business difficulties occurred, Lynn cried and screamed at her partner for as long as he would listen, and then she screamed some more.

About six months after Lynn was out of the business, she was diagnosed as having lymphoma, and about six months after that she came to The Wellness Community. But even one year later, after hours of discussion with her participant group (a psychotherapeutic group that meets weekly) about the effect her anger might be having on her immune system, there was still no way to have a conversation with Lynn that didn't end up with her complaining about her ex-partner. She was obsessed. And that was her immune-depressing condition until the day she died. She just couldn't let it go.

With all that in mind, I will now discuss some methods Lynn could have used to re-form her negative emotions. For that purpose, let's assume that, using the methods suggested in Chapters 5 and 6, you have become aware of an unpleasant emotion in your life, have tracked down its cause—the stressor—and have determined that, for some reason, the stressor can't be altered. So, you must find another way to deal with that state of affairs. The method suggested here is to *attempt* to adjust your reaction to the stressor so that you don't feel the hurt, anger, or shame as intensely as you have been. Here's how to try to do that.

Determine whether your reaction to the stressor is realistic and appropriate.

Start by describing your reaction to the stressor to yourself, to a friend, or to a group, being as objective as possible. When you do this, go into detail and be specific, but omit any drama and pathos; concentrate on the stressor. Don't let your emotions confuse the issue. Ask yourself questions like those set out below. If you are objective and stick to it long enough, the answers to these and other pertinent questions will quite likely become apparent.

1. *What actually is your concern?*
That question is often difficult to answer, although the answer may
seem obvious at first. Consider the mother who wanted her son to
become a physician like his father, and was worried sick (notice
the phrase "worried *sick*") because he was dropping out of school
to become a wood-carver. When asked why she was so anxious to
have her son follow in his father's footsteps, she replied that she
wanted him to be happy. We know, and she knew, that it's quite
possible he would have been miserable as a physician and happy as
a wood-carver. So what was it she was really afraid of? The
possibilities are endless and cry out for examination.

2. *Is your worry, hurt, shame based on current events or is it based on your
   prior experiences?*
An example of the latter reaction is Jenny, who expects that every
man will leave her, because when she was a child, her father left her
for two weeks every month in his job as a traveling salesman and
she always thought it was her fault. Jenny's present pervasive
suspicion that all men will eventually leave her has nothing to do
with the current situation.

3. *If what you are worried about takes place, how badly will you be hurt,
   if at all?*
There is, of course, the possibility that your anxiety is realistic and
that the results will be as severe as you anticipate. However, very often an unemotional consideration of the future will unveil a much
less dire possibility. If you believe you need that man (or woman), as
the song says, more than life itself, you will always be afraid that you
will be left and that life will no longer be worth living. But when
you learn that you don't *need* that person but only *want* her (or him),
and that life will go on even without the person—it always does—
the fear changes to something much less drastic.

4. *How likely is it that what you are worried about will take place?*
It's unrealistic, for example, for a student who has always received
all A's to worry about flunking out.

5. *Are you overreacting?*

6. *Is there a more reasonable way for you to react?*

7. *Is your reaction reasonable and rational?*

Asking yourself these sorts of questions can be an important exercise. If you become aware that your reaction to a particular stressor is neither realistic, appropriate, nor based on current facts, the reaction will automatically disappear without any effort on your part, to be replaced by a more realistic and appropriate response. I know this is hard to believe, but read on.

If you see an uncaged tiger, it's realistic to be afraid it will bite you. However, when you are sure that the tiger has been drugged and has neither teeth nor claws, that fear will disappear. And that's just the point. If you are afraid or worried about something you believe can hurt you, that fear will vanish if you find out that it *can't* hurt you; that the hurt, if it comes, cannot be severe; or that it is very unlikely to happen.

Embarking on this quest for clarity about your reactions will take work, patience, courage, and a willingness to hear observations that may often surprise and sometimes distress you. But learning that your reaction is unrealistic and hard on your immune system may be an important part of your fight for recovery.

Limit, if you can, the duration of the unpleasant emotion.

The question is, how long you are going to permit this unpleasant emotion to continue depressing your immune system? I have heard Wellness Community participants answer this question with another one: How long should we despair over any hurt—no matter how severe? The question becomes more demanding when the strength of your immune system is part of the equation. And for this act of will, I have observed that a determination not to permit the loss or hurt to go on forever seems to have a beneficial effect. Not easy. Not easy at all.

As I considered this question, I became aware that I had no specific advice to give as to how to "limit the duration of the unpleasant emotion," and neither did my colleagues. It then became clear that this was exactly the type of problem that might be best addressed by using the "act as if" method described in Chapter 8 and the Directed Visualization method discussed in Chapter 9.

Control the intensity of the unpleasant emotion resulting from a current situation.

Once again, we must agree before we start that there are those unpleasant emotions that are realistic and, for the most part, unchangeable. However, there are those that can and should be changed. To consider this issue, it's necessary to ask if there really are degrees of unpleasant emotions—and there are. The hurt you feel when your friend doesn't invite you to a party is much less than the hurt of finding that your loved one loves someone else. The fear you feel that it will rain on the football game does not compare with the anxiety as to what the doctor will say after looking at the X rays.

The thrust of this section then is the advice that you make the effort to react less dramatically to those situations that are not that serious, although, at first blush, they may appear so.

Let's go back to Lynn, the entrepreneur who was "kicked out" of the business by her partner, and assume that what she said was factual, that she was unfairly treated. Is it reasonable for her to base her whole life on her hatred for her partner and her distress at being treated unfairly? Do you believe that the degree of emotional travail being suffered should have been ameliorated? Your answer to those questions will give you some clue as to how you deal with similar affairs in your life. Is every slight, hurt, and disappointment more than you can bear? Is every unpleasantness a "big deal"?

Those are the questions you might try to answer, and I believe this can only be done if the troublesome situation is isolated and looked at with the most objectivity you can muster.

As an example of how that is done, consider Leslie, a fifty-two-year-old single woman with breast cancer, who has a job she can't afford to quit because of the medical insurance it provides. The job, however, includes a domineering and unpleasant supervisor. Many nights, Leslie went home with her stomach in knots because of the supervisor, and every morning Leslie felt that she was walking into a combat zone. Leslie tried to discuss the situation with her supervisor, to no avail—nothing changed.

Then, with her friends at The Wellness Community, Leslie found a method she could use that might work. In discussions, her groupmates tried to isolate some specific interactions between Leslie and her supervisor. This was not an easy task. Leslie unconsciously introduced other difficulties of her life into the discussion. She found it difficult to isolate her supervisor from the other problems in her life. And of course, in real life, total isolation cannot take place. But for discussion, it helps. During such discussions, Leslie learned that she saw herself as a weak and helpless child being bullied by an all-powerful persecutor rather than as an adult whose job required her to interact with an unpleasant superior. From that she recognized that, like almost everyone else in the world, she had a job that included some aspects not to her liking. She now reports that she faces every day with those thoughts in mind and she doesn't hate her supervisor as much—she isn't as angry and frustrated all the time. Though this is not a complete solution, the point is that Leslie did something to minimize the unpleasant reaction. She did not just passively accept the immune system–depressing state of siege she was in. That's the suggestion for controlling the intensity of a reaction—do something! Sometimes just directing your attention to the situation in your most objective mode will have a positive effect. And if the situation is of an interpersonal nature, ask yourself—"Can I forgive?" If it was your fault—"Can I atone? Can I apologize?" It's all-important—it's part of your fight for recovery.

Control the intensity of the unpleasant emotion resulting from a tragedy.

As we start this section, we might ask ourselves if we really believe it's possible to limit the reaction to a tragedy such as the loss of a child or spouse. This task is made even more difficult if we try to do it alone. Use your friends as a sounding board. What you are seeking to learn is what action you can take that will decrease the intensity of your unpleasant emotion. You are looking for a method that is unique to you and your personality and your situation. The message of psychotherapist Viktor Frankl, who wrote about his experiences in a Nazi concentration camp in his book *Man's Search For Meaning*, was that the one thing they can't take away from us—over which we have the ultimate control—is our ability to decide how we will react to any situation. The message here is perhaps not to fight the fates but to determine how you will react to the cards dealt to you. That's what a Patient Active does.

Finally, I would suggest again that even if you feel like continuing to grieve about an unhappy, unchangeable event and you believe that such continued grieving is not healthy, you can "act as if" you have accepted the loss and are no longer upset about it or you can try Directed Visualization to intervene between the grief and the resulting negative physical reactions. These methods are discussed in the next two chapters.

CHAPTER 8

∽

How to "Act As If"

For the purpose of this chapter I am assuming that you have become aware of a continuing unpleasant emotion, have determined its cause—the stressor—have taken steps to modify the situation without success, have determined that your reaction is realistic and appropriate, and still the problem continues and, for practical reasons, cannot be escaped. Now is the time you might try the "act as if" method.

The "act as if" technique has two steps: (1) choosing the reaction you believe will be in your best interests, and (2) after you have chosen the reaction, *acting as if* that is the way you feel, even if you don't. Don't forget that the purpose of all this is to prevent unpleasant emotions from suppressing your immune system.

As to step one, most "events" present us with two options: we can react rationally—that is, we can look at our options and choose to react in a way we believe to be in our best interests—or we can react reflexively—automatically, never considering the alternatives. Unfortunately, most people react reflexively most of the time. Usually that's not harmful, because most decisions are inconsequential. However, when those reflexive reactions provoke constant negative emotions, it becomes important, particularly for you as a cancer patient, to consider healthier ways of reacting.

When you know what the better way is, you can force yourself to act in this preferred way, even though it's not comfortable. That's *acting as if*. If you *act as if* long enough and consistently enough, soon this new way of responding will be the way you act

naturally. I hasten to add that choosing what is best for you can be, and often is, based on feelings of love, charity, and compassion; I am certainly not suggesting hedonism. I also want to be clear that this is not an easy matter or one that happens overnight. It takes consistency and perseverance.

The experience of Nadine illustrates how the "act as if" concept works and how it can be used to intervene between stress and the physical reaction to that stress.

In discussions with other cancer patients at The Wellness Community, Nadine, who had lymphoma, realized she had been a "doormat" for her husband and two children for the fifteen years of their marriage—that what they wanted always took priority over what she wanted. Nadine had always reacted to every demand from her family with a "Yes, dear." Whenever her son wanted a ride, she complied, no matter what her plans were. When she was invited to attend a function she would have enjoyed, she always refused the invitation if it would keep her from preparing the dinner her family expected. Because of her training and background, it had never occurred to her that a "good" wife and mother had any alternative.

When Nadine became aware of the doormat quality of her life, she also realized that a part of her was constantly angry at her family's insensitivity to her needs. Then, she decided that it would diminish her anger and be healthier if the stressor—her relationship with her family—evolved into a situation where she was treated as a wife and mother rather than a maid and chauffeur. She had taken the first step. She had chosen the reaction that would be best for her.

The next step was to find a way to make that happen. Nadine tried the first method. She told her husband and children of her anger and asked them to be more considerate of her needs and desires. They tried, but because of inertia and habit, not much changed. And after several months Nadine saw that the first option had failed. Nadine's next step was to *act as if* standing up for her own self-interest was what she felt like doing.

After fifteen years of marriage and a lifetime of compliance, acting as if her own needs and pleasures were important was a difficult change for Nadine. It was made even harder because her family unconsciously resisted her efforts. She was often tempted to give in. However, she persevered, acting as if assertiveness and reasonable self-interest were natural for her.

Here is how Nadine handled situations as they arose: She has plans for an afternoon and her son asks her to drive him to a friend's house, which would ruin her afternoon. Her automatic reaction would be to comply. But with her newfound resolution and in order to accomplish her stated purpose, instead of meekly acquiescing she says something like, "How would it be if I went to my meeting first and took you to your friend's house later?" That reply, after years of being a compliant mother, often triggered a scene—but Nadine stood up to it. And of course, this type of situations with her children and her husband took place day after day after day. Eventually, however, considering her own desires as well as those of others became Nadine's natural reaction, and after a while, Nadine's family started to understand her new position, and their unreasonable requests became less and less frequent. In the process, her anger started to subside, taking some of the pressure off her immune system.

Certainly Nadine took a risk that her family would become alienated and that she would then be faced with returning to her old ways or making a new life for herself. Luckily, Nadine never had to make that choice. The whole family benefited from her newfound assertiveness. Nadine has now been in complete remission for several years, and when I last spoke to her she confided to me that her interaction with her husband—her children are grown—has changed completely. She says it is now based on mutual consideration. She considers that new relationship a benefit of cancer.

Take a moment to examine your own life—either with a group, with a friend, or alone—to see if you can detect any constantly recurring stressor. This can be a difficult assignment. It took Nadine quite a while to admit to herself that she resented her family's insensitivity to her needs. But once she did, it presented

her with the opportunity to actively decide what action she
wanted to take, instead of reacting reflexively. What a wonderful
feeling of freedom and power!

I say again that "acting as if" is not easy, it takes perseverance,
and it doesn't always work. But it's part of your fight for recovery,
and thus is worth the time and effort. And remember, if it doesn't
work for you, that doesn't mean you didn't do it right. It only
means it didn't work.

CHAPTER 9

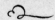

How to Use Directed Visualization

In this chapter, I suggest that you use Directed Visualization, a specific form of meditation (there are a great many forms), to minimize the physical reaction to unpleasant emotions. However, please know that I recommend that everyone—well or ill—use Directed Visualization, or some type of meditation, once or twice a day. It is an effective and easy-to-use tool to reverse the physical reactions to an unpleasant emotion, to reduce pain, and to relax and feel better. It is helpful for everyone, but specifically for cancer patients since it reduces pain and may take some pressure off of the immune system.

The full text of the twenty-minute Directed Visualization technique we recommend appears in Appendix 4. As you'll see, the first ten minutes are devoted to the attempt to enhance the immune system and the second ten minutes are designed to "aim" the healing power of the body at the cancer or the pain. You can read the text onto a tape and use it whenever you want to.

MINIMIZING THE EFFECT UNPLEASANT EMOTIONS HAVE ON THE BODY

Suppose Frank is the owner of a business that's been on the verge of bankruptcy for the last three years, and if he's going to be able to save it at all, it will take three more years of hard work. He knows that if he makes one mistake, that's the end of his business. He can't change the stressor unless he quits, and he doesn't want to do that. He can't change his attitude toward it or "act as if" he doesn't care because if he does the business will certainly fail. Therefore, unless he does something about it, his body is going to be in the immune-suppressing reaction to the stress for the next three years. What should he do? What should you do if you find yourself in a similar situation?

One thing you can do is involve yourself in Directed Visualization, which is a combination of the relaxation techniques described in *The Relaxation Response,* by cardiologist Herbert Benson, M.D., and an attempt to direct the healing power of the body to the area that needs it most. Although both components of Directed Visualization are discussed in this chapter, for more detailed information I highly recommend Dr. Benson's book.

When most people hear words like Directed Visualization they immediately picture a Yogi sitting in the lotus position in a dimly lit, incense-filled room. Furthermore, they assume that the Yogi must have great knowledge, must have suffered and studied extensively and devoted his life to this practice.

But the technique suggested here has no connection with religion, mysticism, the occult, or the exotic. It is an effective, pragmatic method of relaxation that can have a significant beneficial effect on the immune system. It does not take any great skill, practice, or knowledge. Anyone can do it, and there is no way you can do it wrong. No matter how you perform it, it will have some beneficial effect on your immune system. Finally, be assured that once you generally understand the purpose and the simple method described here, there is nothing more anyone can teach you that you won't learn just by continuing to meditate.

Just because this technique is easy to do and not terribly time-consuming, don't be fooled into believing it's not worth doing. Many Patients Active consider Directed Visualization one of the key elements of their fight for recovery. One participant, in describing his bout with cancer, said:

"I also involved myself in Directed Visualization. I really think it's critical. I did it twice a day for a year. And if you ask me whether I believe the mind has power over the body to cure things that are wrong with it, I would tell you that I do. And whether it does or doesn't is almost irrelevant. I thought it was helping me, so I felt good about it. I felt I was in control—that I was going to be victorious.

I think people with cancer who don't visualize are missing the boat, because visualization costs nothing, has no bad side effects, and it makes you feel good even if it doesn't cure cancer—which it might. I don't understand people who don't use every tool available."

THE EFFECTS OF DIRECTED VISUALIZATION

As we know, unpleasant emotions evoke physical reactions which depress the immune system. *It has been scientifically proven that meditation reverses the physical effects of those unpleasant emotions.* Do not pass over that sentence lightly—meditation reverses the physical effects of unpleasant emotions. One of the effects of Directed Visualization is that when you do it your immune system becomes stronger. Dr. Benson's description of the results of his research is the basis for the above assertion. He says: "Because the fight-or-flight response [the body's physical reaction to stress, more explicitly described in Part IV, Question 4]) and the Relaxation Response are in opposition, one counteracts the effect of the other. This is why we feel that the Relaxation Response is of such import, for with its regular use it will offset the harmful effects of the inappropriate elicitation of the fight-or-flight response."

What the sentence says is that meditation minimizes or vitiates the harmful physical effects of stress. For this reason, I cannot emphasize too strongly my belief that you should do some form of meditation once or twice a day while you are fighting to recover.

Some people may be concerned about the potential side effects of meditation. I have never seen or heard of any, and as Dr.

Benson says, "We have noted no [unpleasant side effects] in people who elicit the Relaxation Response daily for ten to twenty minutes."

The second half of Directed Visualization is directed at "aiming" the enhanced power of the immune system at the cancer. No one knows whether that works or not, but it certainly generates a feeling of control over the situation.

Certainly no one, as yet, knows whether Directed Visualization works to reduce the size of a tumor or enhance the possibility of recovery. However, we do know that it makes people feel better, brings about the Relaxation Response, sometimes reduces pain, and returns some control over life to the individuals who practice it.

Most people who have used Directed Visualization enjoy it—look forward to it. They report that it gives them a feeling of participation in the fight for recovery and some control over their lives, and rather paradoxically, at the same time also results in a feeling of serenity and peacefulness. They also report, with deep feeling, that they are certain that it has *some* beneficial results, if only psychological. Hopefully, it will have the same effect on you.

CHAPTER 10

How to Enhance Pleasant Emotions

I have no tricks, but I know that there are two steps you can take which can have wonderful results. First, rid yourself of the myth that, because of the diagnosis, there is no longer a place for joy, gladness, or pleasure in your life. Second, you should know that if you involve yourself in the search for a higher quality of life you will probably find it. I also know that being happy is better than being sad, and because stress depresses the immune system, the higher the quality of life the greater the possibility of recovery. What a wonderful two-way parlay!

So first, let's nullify, abrogate, get rid of the belief that cancer patients must give up all hope for love, joy, fun, laughter, accomplishment, striving, and all other happy feelings. It's just not so! I know hundreds of cancer patients who live full and complete lives within the context of the illness. The participants and ex-participants of The Wellness Community with whom I discussed the contents of this book tell me it's not so, and they were unanimous and enthusiastic in suggesting that I tell you to go out and have as much fun and enjoyment as you can.

Listen to what these cancer patients and ex–cancer patients are saying to you. They are telling you that you can do it, because they have done it, and in addition, they are suggesting that you pursue happiness, joy, and fun for the same reason you accept chemo or radiation or surgery—as part of your battle against cancer. They also gleefully remind you that the only side effects of an assertive search for happiness is an improved quality of life. Whoopee!

I know that what these people are saying is true. Since 1982 cancer patients have been telling me how cancer has changed their lives—how they have been able to stop and smell the roses, how they have improved their relationships with their loved ones, how they have learned to enjoy their work and the other everyday aspects of their lives. What they are saying, of course, is that as they went through life before cancer, they took those elements of their lives for granted as if they would never lose them, and now that losing them is a possibility, they are savoring each moment. Seems to me a better way to live, sick or well.

If you don't believe that people with cancer can still enjoy themselves you ought to come to a Wellness Community Joke Fest. There's one at every Wellness Community at least twice each year. A Joke Fest is an evening when a large group of Wellness Community participants come together and try to outdo each other by telling some of the worst jokes you have ever heard. I have been to many of these Joke Fests and I tell you that the room is always filled with gales of laughter brought on by the quality of the jokes. Don't tell any of those joke tellers that the time for laughter is over!

Gilda Radner was always the star of the Joke Fests she was in. Not because she was famous but because she was funny—very funny—and because she wanted to live life to the fullest. Gilda told me several times that when she heard the diagnosis, she was sure that the times of fun and being funny were over for her. I was thrilled when she said that it was in a meeting at The Wellness Community that she lost the depression she was feeling and real- ized that life could be fun again, that she could be funny again, and that life was worth living. When we had those conversations, Gilda was still under treatment but she was filled with energy and joy. What Gilda learned at The Wellness Community was her wake-up call to come back to living life. This can be yours.

The subject of laughter is more complex than most of us

realize. But there is one aspect of laughter that everyone agrees with: laughter is healthy—it's good for you. But as we consider the benefits of laughter, it's important to be aware of the following statement made by my mentor Norman Cousins, whom I will discuss in more detail shortly. Here's what he said: "Laughter in and of itself cannot cure nor prevent cancer, but laughter as a part of the full range of positive emotions including hope, love, faith, a strong will to live and determination can be a significant part of the total fight for recovery."

Here's a cancer patient's view of laughter. Dan, who had prostate cancer, was asked by the host of a comedy TV show, "Do you believe that laughter really does you any good—not because other people have told you that it should, but because you have experienced it?"

I know laughter is good for me. I don't know if it is helping me get better, but it makes me feel better—not only mentally but physically as well—and it takes my mind off my own situation. Life and its pleasures have become very real to me and I know just how important it is to enjoy each enjoyable minute. So when something strikes me as laughable, I laugh. I want to be conscious of every joyful part of life.

Before cancer, I only paid attention to the problems of life, the need and difficulty of making a living, maintaining relationships, and getting ahead. The frustrating and hurtful incidents were the ones I related to my friends when they said, "How are things?" Occasionally, we talked about the good times, but it seems to me that what I did the most . . . was complain, and I took the pleasant and joyful parts of life as routine and as my due.

That's all different now. Now I accentuate the positive and eliminate the negative . . . Most importantly, I make sure that I am aware of the good times when they come along. So when something is funny, I laugh; and that reinforces my certainty that life is good.

Another booster of the benefits of laughter is Lee Berk, Ph.D., of Loma Linda Hospital, who conducted a study which reinforces the theory that laughter enhances the immune system. Berk hooked five healthy medical students to a blood machine and took blood from them every five minutes while they were watching a thirty-minute funny film. The students roared with laughter; I was there. Berk reported in scientific jargon that ". . . laughter may be an antagonist to the classical stress response." What that means is that laughter enhanced the immune system. Studies by William Fry, M.D., of Stanford University and Patti Ekman, Ph.D., of the University of California, San Francisco, tested the immune systems of participants before and after laughter or smiling, and both concluded that "laughter/humor resets the immune system."

Now that we know that pleasant emotions enhance the immune system, let's get on with taking affirmative action to enhance pleasant emotions. This part takes effort, but it's worth it. Norman Cousins, who recovered from a most serious illness, is a perfect example of the benefits of laughter and consciously taking action to improve the quality of life.

In 1979 Cousins—then the editor of the *Saturday Review* and immediately before his death an adjunct professor at the UCLA School of Medicine as well as honorary chairman of The Wellness Community's Board of Trustees, wrote *Anatomy of an Illness*, published by Norton. In that book, Cousins described his fight with and recovery from ankylosing spondylitis, which he described as "a disintegration of the connective tissue of the spine—a particularly painful, debilitating, and sometimes fatal disease." Here's what he wrote:

It was easy enough to hope, love, and have faith, but what about laughter? Nothing is less funny than being flat on your back with all the bones in your spine and joints hurting. A systematic program was indicated. A good place to begin, I thought, was with amusing movies. Allen Funt, producer of the spoofing television program "Candid Camera," sent films of some of his "CC" classics, along with a motion-picture projector. The nurse was instructed in its use. We were able to get our hands on some old Marx Brothers films. We pulled down the blinds and turned on the machine.

It worked. I made the joyous discovery that ten minutes of genuine belly laughter had an anesthetic effect and would give me at least two hours of pain-free sleep. When the pain-killing effects of the laughter wore off, we would switch on the motion-picture projector again, and not infrequently, it would lead to another pain-free sleep interval. Sometimes the nurse read to me out of a trove of humor books. Especially useful were E. B. and Katherine White's *Subtreasury of American Humor* and Max Eastman's *The Enjoyment of Laughter*.

How scientific was it to believe that laughter—as well as the positive emotions in general—was affecting my body chemistry for the better? If laughter did in fact have a salutary effect on the body's chemistry, it seemed at least theoretically likely that it would enhance the system's ability to fight the inflammation. (It seemed to be working.) I was greatly elated by the discovery that there is a physiologic basis for the ancient theory that laughter is good medicine.

Although Cousins's description of his laughter experiment was brief, many people interpreted the main message of the book to be that laughter had "cured" him. Cousins called that interpretation of his statements "an absurd notion." No scientific professional has ever argued that laughter can cure cancer or any other disease. However, as part of the total range of positive emotions, laughter may have a salutary effect on the recovery process.

There is a major difference between taking assertive action to pursue happiness, as I am suggesting here, and accepting chemo, surgery, and radiation. In taking chemo "they" do it to you. In seeking happiness you have to do it yourself, and to some people that's easy—they just continue to enjoy life as they did before, within the restrictions of the illness. To others it's very difficult.

Perhaps you're saying to yourself, "I don't want to do that. I have every right to be resentful. Look what happened to me." And it's difficult to disagree with that. You do have a right to be resentful. And if that's what feels comfortable for you, then do it and don't let anyone talk you out of it. That may sound like a manipulation—but I promise you it's not. My experience has taught me that there are some wonderful and brave people who have come to an accommodation with cancer which is satisfactory for them. You might consider whether you are one of them.

And there are other reasons people give themselves for giving up the search for happiness which we should discuss to determine if any of them are applicable to you. I have heard cancer patients say that they are just too ill from the cancer or its treatment to try to enjoy life, and I'm sure that's true. But isn't it also true that even with the most dire prognosis and the most severe treatment, there is still time off, there is still time to try to enjoy life? That's what I've been told and I have watched many cancer patients take that route.

Another reason for being passive about seeking enjoyment is that the fear of the future is so pervasive as to leave no room for any other emotion. But I have seen so many people convert that dread into an energetic search for a higher quality of life that I am sure it can be done. One of my great pleasures is watching that metamorphosis happen. There is no greater joy than to watch faces light up and hope become almost palpable. I hope you experience that renewed will to live.

At this time, a short discussion of that phrase "the will to live" is in order. A few truisms will be helpful. First, the will to live is a gauge of the quality of life. Think about that. Isn't it true that the higher the quality of life the greater the will to live? Second, it's also true that the greater the will to live the more likely the recovery. I have heard many physicians make that statement. When you add those statements together, you come to the conclusion that the higher the quality of life the more likely the recovery. Here's how that works:

The higher the quality of life the greater the will to live.

The greater the will to live the more likely the recovery.

Therefore, the higher the quality of life the more likely the recovery. What a wonderful reason to strive for a higher quality of life!

As I write about seeking enjoyment as part of the fight for recovery, I am reminded of a situation where I was talking to a Wellness Community participant about the benefits of affirmatively seeking to enjoy life. As we spoke I noticed a look of distress come over his face, and I asked him if anything I said had caused it. And it had. He said that I was placing too much pressure on him—that it was too tough to go out and seek pleasure, that he had never done that and he couldn't do it now. And for him, he was right. The search for happiness was too much for him at that time—maybe later.

So let's be clear here. Whatever you do or don't do is perfect for you. These are not admonitions. These are suggestions which I *hope* will have a positive effect on your immune system and I *believe* will improve the quality of your life. Nothing more. Many people, perhaps most, never affirmatively seek fun—they wait until it comes to them. So for them, and maybe for you, affirmatively seeking happiness is as difficult as jumping six feet into the air. And if it is, you can try it or not as you wish. It's your choice.

If, however, you want to try to enhance pleasant emotions, I'm going to suggest that you make a list—a list of what you liked to do—what made you happy—before the diagnosis, and then, one by one, decide if you can still do them, and if not why not. Ask yourself the following questions: "Can I still do it? Can I still do any part of it? Can I do it alone? If it needs another person or other people—are they there for me? What is preventing me from doing it? Can I overcome that obstacle?"

Also, use the Quality of Life charts described in Chapter 6 and make a list of those occasions, activities, interactions which, now that you know how important each day is, give you pleasure. Actually, this is a wonderful method for bringing to your consciousness those aspects of your life that were previously underappreciated. Some have called this a benefit of cancer.

With the list in hand, start making decisions about what you can and want to do and what you can't and don't want to do.

So, give yourself permission to laugh and enjoy life, and make sure that your family and friends permit and help you to laugh. Most well people believe that the only way to act around a cancer patient is downcast, unhappy, and sympathetic. Under those circumstances, it's easy to play the part of the doomed object of pity and give up all laughter and fun. But don't do it—and don't let them do it to you. Your family and friends don't mean to get in the way of your enjoyment of life. They just need to be educated about what you need and want. Tell them you want them to act with you as they did before the illness. Point out that you want to enjoy life.

Laughter and being involved with other people's lives—as well as going on with love, fun, and involvement in your own life—is important. The statement "It's fun to laugh" may be redundant, but it's meaningful.

III

SPECIFIC METHODS TO FIGHT FOR RECOVERY

CHAPTER 11

⌒ℓ⌒

Hope—Regain It, Maintain It, and Sustain It

A few definitions will be helpful for this discussion. Hope consists of three elements: (1) a desire that an event will take place, (2) the *possibility* that that event will occur, and (3) the belief that you will be pleased if it does. Hopelessness, on the other hand, consists of only two elements: (1) a desire that an event will take place and (2) the belief that no matter what you do, there is no possibility that the event will occur. Thus you see that hopelessness always includes a feeling of helplessness. And in most cases of cancer neither hopelessness nor helplessness is realistic, although the myths about cancer would fool you into believing otherwise. As a matter of fact, in the great majority of cases it's unreasonable and unrealistic *not* to have hope.

Hopelessness, from another point of view, is the certainty that what you want to happen will not happen. There is a certain arrogance in such a feeling. How can you be so certain about anything that will take place in the future?

Lack of hope is a serious matter for the cancer patient. The literature is replete with information indicating that loss of hope is one of the three most debilitating psychological problems cancer patients face, along with unwanted aloneness and loss of control. The belief that the situation is hopeless—that you are doomed—results in lethargy, listlessness, and passive acceptance of what is perceived as inevitable. Why would you, or anyone else, fight if there is no hope for recovery? Can you think of anything more melancholy, any emotion more depressing? As far as the fight for recovery goes, hope is good—hopelessness is bad. I can't think of one redeeming feature of hopelessness. Few researchers have better summarized the effect hope can have on recovery than Fred O. Henker, M.D., a professor of psychiatry at the University of Arkansas. At a meeting of the American Psychiatric Association, after describing various aspects of the process of recovery from illness, Henker concluded with this pithy statement: "Whether we acknowledge the influence of hope or not, it's real, and it may even determine the life or death outcome of the patient." I have yet to meet a physician who does not agree with that statement.

So hope for recovery is important to you, and it might be helpful for you to look inside right now. On a scale of 1 to 10—10 being absolute certainty that the outcome will be as you want it to be—do you feel hopeless?

If you are not sure, you might ask someone who knows you well and you trust questions like the following:

- Have I been using words that indicate I believe I am doomed?
- Have I been acting as if I believe there is no hope?
- Does it appear that I am drawing away from those I care about and who care about me?
- Do I appear more listless and lethargic than usual? (Of course, your physical condition may play a part in this answer.)

If the answers indicate to you that you have less hope than you would like, read on. If it appears that you are brimming with hope, unless you are curious go to another chapter.

There are only a few reasons for the feelings of hopelessness. One is based on the myths about cancer—that everyone who is diagnosed with cancer dies of it. We can dispense with that myth by, once again, citing the data published by the American Cancer Society in its 1994 bulletin, *Cancer Facts and Figures*. That prestigious organization indicates that 40 to 50 percent of all people who have cancer recover from the illness and that there are eight million Americans alive today who have a history of cancer. At least half of these eight million are considered completely recovered, meaning that they have no evidence of the illness and have the same life expectancy as a person who has never had cancer. Look at those figures again and see that one out of two people recover and that those who recover *have the same life expectancy as if they had never had cancer.* In the 1930s one in five survived. In the 1940s one in four. In the 1960s one in three, and now, using all the figures available, it's one in two. So your feeling that the outcome is assured is not supported by the facts.

Another factor that can thwart hope is that you know, from one source or another, that everyone who has your type of cancer dies of it. That's just not true. I believe your physician will tell you that there is no type of cancer that does not have some recovery rate. Some are better than others, but every cancer has a recovery rate—so the outcome of your cancer is not certain. And in the situation where only one out of a hundred patients survives the illness you have, isn't it reasonable to hope that you are that one? Of course it is.

Another cause for hopelessness is that you feel in your bones (intuitively) that your time is up. This, of course, is the most dangerous because it is based on nothing you can refute, and can become a self-fulfilling prophecy. I suggest that you talk to someone about that to see where it comes from.

Now let's discuss some actions you can take to eliminate or at least minimize that melancholy emotion. I suggest you avoid stress by using the methods in Chapters 5 through 10, that you meet or become aware of other or ex–cancer patients as suggested in Chapters 18 and 19, that you keep up your social contacts as described in Chapters 15, 16, and 17, that you use hopeful and optimistic words about the illness as suggested in Chapter 25, and that you make plans for the future as suggested in Chapter 28. Those methods restore hope.

FALSE HOPE

There is no way to examine hope in a cancer patient's life without recognizing the possibility of false hope. When I decided to start The Wellness Community, some people argued that such a program would foster false hope. Frankly, at first I gave these thoughts serious consideration, but then I realized that these critics erroneously believed that our program would tell cancer patients we "guaranteed" they would get well if they followed our advice. Nothing could be farther from the truth. We have always known there is no such thing as a sure cure. Promises that "if you do what we tell you, you *will* get well" are not messages of false hope; they're either fraud or stupidity.

Even Norman Cousins was concerned about creating false hope when he wrote *Anatomy of an Illness* describing his fight against a life-threatening illness. He said, "I have not written in any detailed way about my illness . . . largely because I was fearful of creating false hopes in other persons similarly afflicted."

Cousins was worried that people who had the same disease would believe that if they indulged in large doses of laughter and vitamin C, as he did, they would be *guaranteed* recovery. He took great pains in his book not to create the illusion that he was making any promises of recovery, while emphasizing that there is always room for hope.

Actually, there is no such thing as false hope. All clichés have some truth in them, and the pertinent cliché here is, "Where there's life, there's hope."

Up to this point, we have discussed hope only in terms of complete recovery. But even for patients who have accepted the inevitability of something other than complete recovery, there can be hope for joy, love, and involvement in life. Just as life does not end with the diagnosis of cancer, life does not end when the possibility of recovery becomes remote. Life goes on as long as life goes on.

Finally, although no one can promise complete recovery, hope is there for the taking. And with hope comes an improved quality of life, which is a reasonable goal in itself.

CHAPTER 12

≈

Control—Take It Back

Unless handled with care, loss of control and the resulting feeling of helplessness can be serious problems to the cancer patient. They can lead to a giving-up behavior and loss of the will to live, two potent negative stressors. Later in this chapter, I will describe several studies on both humans and animals which indicate just how debilitating loss of control can be.

For that reason, it is my belief that efforts to retain, maintain, and regain as much control as is reasonable should be given high priority in the cancer patient's fight for recovery. The thrust of this chapter is directed to that effort. However, I am also going to advise that this be done with caution so that you do not bite off more than you can chew. Finally, with full knowledge that when cancer is the diagnosis, some control of one's life must be relinquished, I am going to suggest that the yielding of control that cannot be retained be accepted with composure and equanimity, so that the loss of control does not in itself become the stressor.

ACTIONS YOU CAN TAKE TO MAINTAIN, REGAIN, OR SUSTAIN CONTROL

STEP ONE:
Determine just how much control you have given up.
Make a list of the areas of control you have given up—in other

words, what decisions are now made for you that you have always made for yourself and what functions previously performed by you are now performed by others. Treat this list seriously. Be specific about what you have given up. You will probably be surprised to find you have relinquished control where you needn't have.

STEP TWO:
Make a list of what have you given up that you can take back. Be careful here. Don't be too aggressive.

STEP THREE:
Begin taking back control one step at a time, starting with the easy ones. To begin with, you can immediately take control of one significant part of your life—deciding exactly what you will and won't eat. Reading Chapter 33 may help you make those decisions. You might also suggest to your health care providers that they allow you to make choices about routine matters, such as which arm to take blood from. A Rand Corporation scientist who studied the impact of loss of control on cancer patients came to the conclusion that when patients made choices about daily matters and educated themselves about the illness, they experienced better health and a heightened sense of well-being, as well as less stress and anxiety.

I caution you again, in deciding what areas of control you will take back don't be unreasonable. If you take on more than you can handle, you can impede the recovery process and make life unbearable for those around you. What are you to do now? Up to this point, you have been counseled to take back control, to make choices, to choose between alternatives—all of which are aggressive, affirmative suggestions. But now you've been urged to use caution and reasonableness. Thus you see that being a Patient Active requires that you walk a fine line—aggressively taking back control while not biting off more than you can chew.

Combining these two seemingly contradictory guidelines results in the following recommendation: Do everything in your power to accentuate conduct you believe may be conducive to your recovery, and eliminate habits that may be interfering with that process. This advice—obvious, yet often difficult to live up to—takes on its proper importance when you realize that in order to follow it, you must examine reactions that have always been automatic to determine if there is an alternative that might be better for you. Such examination alone—just assessing the prospective behavior to see if it is bad or good for you—can result in your having more control of your life than ever before. It will move the decision-making process from the unconscious to the conscious, from the instinctive to the purposeful, from the reflexive to the deliberate. If you follow these guidelines, you will decide how you want to react to a specific life event based on current facts rather than memories of past experiences. You will decide whether the automatic responses you've always had are healthy or unhealthy. This is a potent way of taking control.

Most people with cancer know only too well the feelings of depression brought on by cancer-related loss of control. A dependence on others after a lifetime of independence and self-sufficiency often provokes such feelings. Routine tasks become monumental undertakings. Those who depended on you in the past have now become those on whom you depend. Almost everything is different. And no matter what you do, all this is likely to continue to some extent until you recover.

Some cancer patients who have lost some control—often temporarily—believe that they have lost *all* control *forever*. They further believe that depression and despair are the only normal reactions to the loss of any control, and that there is nothing they can do to retain or regain control of any part of their lives. They are, for the most part, wrong. Many cancer patients, just like you, have substituted involvement for helplessness and hope for despair, after they realized that they had retained more control than they thought they could, that there are many ways a Patient Active can regain much of the control he or she has given up, and that every cancer patient can learn to accept, with some degree of equanimity, the loss of control he or she can't retain.

At this point, it's important to recall that all negative stress is the result of remembering, experiencing, or anticipating a situation that we believe can harm us either mentally or physically, and *over which we have no control.* If we believe we are in control of a situation—that is, if we can prevent it from harming us physically or mentally—anxiety vanishes. Thus, if I can control the discussion with the boss so he won't fire me, or the confrontation with a robber so he won't hurt me, or the opinions of my friends so they will always respect and admire me, I will have little or no negative stress.

This concept is important because it justifies working so hard to retain control. And just making the effort to retain control—or, after consideration, to concede that there is an area of control that is reasonable to give up—relieves a great deal of anxiety.

Of course, if the "deal" you have made with God or the universe is that life is good only on your terms, and your terms are that you will always be in full control, then you will find any loss of control unacceptable. If, on the other hand, you are aware that the amount of control you have, like everything else in life, ebbs and flows, you can accept the loss of some control with serenity. As philosophers through the ages have said, the ultimate control—how you perceive and react to the loss of control you cannot retain—is yours.

The concept that loss of control can impede the fight for recovery is based on many human and animal studies which I will discuss to reinforce your determination to take back as much control as is reasonable. In one of these human studies a group of healthy males was divided into three groups: (1) those with few life stressors; (2) those with many life stressors who responded with high anxiety (had little control); and (3) those with many life stressors who responded with low anxiety (had much control).

Not surprisingly, the study found that the "many stressors/much control" group had stronger immune systems than the "many stressors/little control" group. What surprised everyone is that the "many stressors/much control" also had stronger immune systems than even the "few stressors" group. Obviously then, it's not the stressors that cause the problem; it's the lack of control that does the harm.

Another human study surveyed a group of fifty-one women who had just taken a test to determine if they had cervical cancer. That study revealed that although the questionnaire was answered before the results were known, 61 percent of the women who felt they had little control over their lives had cancer, while only 24 percent of the women who felt in control of their lives had the illness—more evidence to buttress the belief that the loss of control may play a part in the onset of cancer and therefore can quite possibly affect the recovery process.

Animal studies have been even more conclusive. In one study, three groups of mice were injected with cancer cells. One group was then exposed to electric shocks which they could turn off by touching a bar. A second group was exposed to shocks over which they had no control. The third group received no shocks. The researchers found that the tumor growth in the mice receiving *uncontrollable* shocks was significantly greater than that of the other two groups and that there was no significant difference in tumor growth between the group that received no shocks and the group that received controllable shocks. The researchers concluded that controllable stress is the same as no stress at all, at least as far as the immune system in mice is concerned.

In another study of mice, the test was to determine what the "social" effect on mice would be after a prolonged period of stress over which they had no control. The same three situations were set up—controllable, uncontrollable, and no shocks at all. It was found that at the end of the test the mice with uncontrollable shocks were listless, would not fight for food, and were passive when handled. The mice with shocks they could control were just about the same as those who had no shocks at all—that is, there was no immune system impairment. That means that stress over which they had control had no negative effects. If the same results were attributed to humans, that would mean that stress we can control has no negative effects. I hope that is the case.

On the other hand, if the results of the mice tests were directly referable to humans, it would mean that if we experienced stress over which we had no control, we would invariably experience serious negative consequences. That was the result with the mice. I do not subscribe to that extrapolation. We are not like mice. We can observe the passing scene and make decisions as to what is acceptable and what is not. We can accommodate to uncontrollable stress by accepting it with composure and not letting that loss become a new stressor.

I have watched many cancer patients mature to the point where situations that would have driven them crazy before the diagnosis are now put into a more realistic perspective. How important is it, they ask, that the situation is not developing as they want it to? Is it important enough to cause a traumatic reaction? Those are the types of questions you might ask yourself in relation to the everyday events in your life.

To sum up, here's what we know: You may be able to affect the course of the illness by (1) regaining and sustaining as much control as is reasonable, and (2) by giving up with equanimity rather than rage the loss of control you cannot retain. But do not underestimate or overestimate that statement. We all have a great deal of control, but we are not omnipotent. None of us is in complete control of the final outcome of any situation, particularly the recovery from cancer. While it behooves cancer patients to muster their every resource to respond to life events in the most positive manner, there is no assurance that the outcome will be as hoped. But remember, if the illness does not progress as you want it to, it's not because you didn't do enough or didn't do things well enough. Sometimes the outcome is out of our hands.

I had three teenage daughters, a husband, and colon cancer. We are a very close family. We all live in the same house. I work at home. I am an accountant. When the diagnosis was made, my family came flying to my aid and, being the competent human beings they were, took over all of the functions around the house I previously performed. Somehow, I was delighted. I felt very sorry for myself. After about three months of this, while

I was in treatment but continuing to act as an accountant, my youngest daughter, who was fourteen at the time, called a family meeting and said that she was tired of doing all of the work that was being placed on her, that I looked like I could take back some of the responsibility, and that she wanted me to. The rest of the family looked a little embarrassed, but obviously understood what she was saying. Even I understood. Everything changed then and there, and I believe to my benefit. I started to act like part of the team again and I was once again in control of much of my life. From there, I started to take back more and more activity. I think that was better for me. I know I like me better.

Carrie

CHAPTER 13

⌒⌒

Anger—Find It, Examine It, and Get Rid of It

Before we start, a few facts will set this chapter in context. First, it will be helpful to become aware of the meaning of the words "repress" and "suppress," as I will be making the distinction throughout this chapter. To repress an emotion such as anger is an unconscious act and to suppress it is a conscious act. Second, you may find it hard to believe, but there are people who have no recollection of ever feeling anger. Of course, they have been in situations that have angered them, but they don't even know it. They have repressed it—that is, they have blocked it from their awareness. We have all met people who seem never to become angry—who never lose their temper—who accept everything with calmness. Those are the people I am talking about.

Third, anger is a most powerful and unpleasant immune-depressing emotion. Fourth, if we think about it, we all know that we have two alternatives in regard to anger of which we are aware. We can express it by shouting at the driver of the car that cut in front of us or using the other methods of venting our anger available to us, or we can *suppress* it—that is, consciously refrain from expressing that anger. We all suppress anger many times throughout our daily lives. If we expressed our anger every time we felt it, we would be in constant combat with those around us.

With that information in mind we can discuss anger as it effects a cancer patient. Although there is little hard evidence of a connection between cancer and *unacknowledged* anger, it is a widely accepted, unproven thesis that there is such a connection. The theory is that (1) anger is an unpleasant emotion, (2) that *unacknowledged* anger is a long-term, unpleasant emotion because it will remain until it is expressed, and (3) since we know that long-term, unremitting, unpleasant emotions depress the immune system, we can extrapolate that *unacknowledged* anger is a long-term, unpleasant emotion that depresses the immune system.

On the other hand, if the anger is *acknowledged* and *expressed* or *acknowledged* and *suppressed*, it doesn't seem to be harmful and may even be useful. Therefore, the first aim of the cancer patient, as far as anger is concerned, is to become aware of repressed anger if any there is, and bring it to consciousness where it can be dealt with. The second aim is to consciously choose how to deal with it, either express it or, with full knowledge of all the implications, decide to suppress it. I will first deal with the possibility that you repress anger when it is a reasonable reaction.

ACTIONS YOU CAN TAKE

STEP ONE
Determine if you have repressed anger. The purpose here is to bring any repressed anger to consciousness. Ask yourself if you often find yourself in situations where anger would be a reasonable reaction and it is not the emotion that is evoked in you. Very often, we find, just bringing the possibility of repressed anger to the top of your consciousness will reveal whether or not you are repressing anger. If that sounds like a simple task—believe me, it's not. It takes hard work and dedication, and maybe repressed anger is not there at all. But if you have a hard time remembering when you were angry last, perhaps you might discuss anger with a friend. Ask that friend whether you react to situations with anger when he or she believes anger is called for. You might get some interesting answers. If it doesn't seem to be an overriding emotion—and it

won't for those of us who express anger at the drop of a hat—move on. If, on the other hand, you find that there is more anger than you believe is good for you, read on.

STEP TWO
Get rid of it. There are several methods for dissipating anger you are aware of which have proven quite effective. The first is to confront the anger and discuss it openly with the subject of your anger, if that's possible and reasonable.

The second is to talk about the fury, trying to make some sense of it by attempting to describe it and explain it. Talking it out forces you to put into coherent form the undisciplined and un-bridled emotions running through your mind. Some people at-tempting this approach struggle valiantly but are unable to come up with a series of sentences that make any sense. The frustration of that failure sometimes dissolves into laughter or tears, which somehow places the anger in a new perspective. Others describe their anger so cogently and clearly that for the first time they really understand it and have a better idea of what to do with it. And that can also dissipate anger.

The third approach to freeing oneself from the ravages of unexpressed anger is the screaming, punching method— arranging to be where you can give vent to the fury by scream-ing, punching pillows, stamping your feet, cursing at the object of your hostility, and using every other method of expressing anger you can think of. The purpose is to expel from your mind the hostility that may be suppressing your immune system. While this method does not bring about understanding, it certainly releases tension.

There is another way of expressing anger; unfortunately, it is the most common. In this approach, the cancer patient is not aware he is angry but unconsciously "acts out" by becoming spiteful and antagonistic to everyone around him; the anger leaks out in venom and pettiness. This method doesn't get rid of any-thing but friends and is in every way counterproductive. The release of tension is so slow that it doesn't do anybody any good.

ANGER—PROPERLY USED—
CAN BE BENEFICIAL

A study of women with breast cancer by Martin Abeloff, Ph.D., and Leonard Derogatis, Ph.D., in 1977 found that giving vent to anger was physically beneficial. They wrote, "Women who can express hostility survive metastatic breast cancer longer than non-assertive, compliant women."

In the same vein, Steven Greer, Ph.D., and Tina Morris in 1979 published a report of a five-year study in which they found that "women who had either a 'fighting spirit' or who were absolute deniers have a statistically significant advantage both in disease-free interval and mortality compared to those who are hopeless/helpless or stoic acceptors." And it is women who are hopeless, helpless, and stoic who suppress anger.

From all of the above comes the following advice: Become angry when anger is appropriate. Express that anger when such expression is appropriate. When it is deemed reasonable and prudent to suppress anger—do that with full knowledge of what you are doing and why you are doing it. When it is not appropriate to express your anger, use one of the other methods of getting rid of it. Make sure it just doesn't hang on forever.

One other aspect of anger you might consider is whether you become angry at matters that are actually not that important. Too much anger, even if expressed or otherwise dissipated, is not in your best interest and, to the best of your ability, should be controlled.

EXPRESSED ANGER

Another aspect of anger that deserves attention is that of anger and hostility constantly experienced. For a more complete analysis of that reaction to life and the unhealthy effects of such a personality trait, I refer you to *Anger Kills* by Redford and Virginia Williams.

The authors comment on the health-impairing possibility of constantly felt anger as follows: "This [study] suggests that in addition to contributing to higher death rates via coronary situations, hostility might also be contributing to increased risk of cancer as well."

For the purposes of this section, I will consider the word "hostile" to describe a person who feels anger easily and "anger" to mean the emotion triggered by an event perceived by the individual as anger-provoking. An example of a hostile person is one who when he or she is cut off on a freeway sees that as a reason for immediate and violent anger, while someone less hostile would consider the event a mere annoyance.

If you are a person who feels anger easily and often—too often—you might want to deal with what may be a problem from two points of view: dealing with the immediate anger and taking steps to become less hostile.

The Williamses suggest that when anger is experienced, it is important to determine whether (1) the anger is worth your continued attention, (2) it is justified, and (3) you have an effective response. If the answer to any of those questions is no, they suggest you might take some action to control the anger. They go on to outline seventeen methods of dealing with the immediate situation, including meditation, reasoning with yourself, asserting yourself, and distraction. It is further hypothesized that if you use these anger-controlling methods consistently, your innate hostility may be diminished. That's what we want to happen.

I was twenty-six years old, married for three years, my husband's first novel was selling very well, and along came lymphoma. I was sure I was going to die. But I was not frightened. I was furious and I let everyone know it and I was becoming impossible to live with. Lucky for me I lived near a Wellness Community and my friends in my Participant Group talked with me about my anger often. One day, they decided that the way they would deal with my anger was to agree with me and exaggerate everything I said, and the room became more and more noisy with people agreeing with me that it was my husband's fault and my mother's fault, and the fault of the food I ate and everything else I blamed the illness on. The angrier we all got the noisier it became. Suddenly, after about fifteen minutes, the climax came and we all sat back exhausted. Everything had changed for me. I'm not even sure I can describe the change. I was still angry, but I was calm and determined to do everything I could to get better. I was not out of control. My life was better. I am now in long-term remission and I go for checkups regularly and I'm still worried, but my anger is focused and controllable.

Vivian

CHAPTER 14

❧

Myths About Cancer— Eliminate Them

The myths about cancer are as deeply ingrained in our psyches as the myth about the flatness of the earth once was. They come to us from the highest authorities, and they have actually become a part of us. It's vitally important for you to know that if these myths continue to be your basic belief, they can do much harm. They can inhibit you from consciously taking actions that may benefit your recovery process. They can be the cause of long-term, unremitting unpleasant emotions. They may inhibit your mind/body from automatically performing its self-healing functions. They may become self-fulfilling prophecies, and may make recovery less likely than it might otherwise be. Although these myths and misconceptions are absurd, they stubbornly persist, often transforming cancer from an illness of the body to a disease of the soul.

To understand the methods suggested to get rid of these myths, let's first define "myth." As we use the term, a myth is a community-held belief that proves to be false once the actual facts emerge. For example, people believed for a long time that the earth was flat and that if they ventured too far out to sea, they would fall off. All decisions were based upon that "fact." The world was circumscribed with an imaginary boundary, and traffic and cultural exchange between continents were impossible. The flat-world myth persisted until Columbus disproved it.

The myths about cancer are equally false. Listed below are some of them. Read them carefully and think about them and discuss them with your friends. That's the best way I know to free yourself from their depressing influence. It is my experience that these myths can continue to frighten us only so long as they are vague and undefined, and that they disappear when they are exposed to discussion and analysis.

The advice then is—discuss them with your friends and physician, analyze them, consider them, make fun of them. That's it—make fun of them. Ask yourself questions like, "Do you really believe that cancer is shameful? Why? In heaven's name, why?" Look inside and see how much each myth is a part of your basic belief system. What do you believe your doctor will reply if you ask, "Doctor, am I to blame because I have cancer?"

All of these myths are discussed in this book. And this advice, unlike some of the other advice in the book, is easy to do and won't cause any trouble. Try it!

COMMON MYTHS ABOUT CANCER

1. Cancer is always invincible.
   That's just wrong. I know hundreds and hundreds of ex-cancer patients—many of whom have undergone transplantations, chemo, operations, radiation, nausea, lethargy, etc., etc., and are now living full and complete lives.

2. Life ends with the diagnosis.
   Wrong again. Read Chapter 10 to see just how wrong it is.

3. Cancer is contagious.
   Ask your doctor if that's not a myth.

4. Cancer is shameful.
   There's not much to say about how silly that is.

5. There is nothing the cancer patient can do to help in the fight for recovery.
   This whole book disproves that myth.

6. Once the disease is diagnosed, the cancer patient must turn over all control of his or her life to others.
Same observation as 5.

7. The cancer patient is to blame for the illness.
See Chapter 31.

8. It is the cancer patient's fault if she is not recovering as quickly as she thinks she should.
See Chapter 32.

They're all myths! You don't need them! They get in the way! Get rid of them!

I attended a recent discussion meeting of Wellness Community partici-
pants. One of the questions for discussion was: Why is cancer considered
shameful and embarrassing? All of the participants had cancer and all
admitted that they were, to one degree or another, embarrassed by that fact.
At first, the conversation was as serious as could be. We talked about the
fact that cancer was the modern-day leprosy and that some people believed
that cancer was contagious. But gradually it became obvious just how
ridiculous this particular myth is. As we started to reach for the reasons
behind the myth, we all became increasingly silly, and the meeting ended
with laughter and shouting—all of us trying to prove that the myth was a
fact. From that laughter, we all learned that cancer is no more shameful
than any other illness—that cancer is visited on the rich and the poor, the
young and the old, the educated and the uneducated, the sanitary and the
unsanitary. All of the participants said they had once been ashamed and
embarrassed about having cancer but were no longer. They had lost their
shame when they met others who had or had had cancer and who were not
ashamed or embarrassed by that fact, and when they learned to discuss
cancer openly instead of in whispers.

Leonard

CHAPTER 15

Don't Be Reclusive

Human relations are desperately important to both our mental and physical well-being. The fact is that social isolation, the lack of human companionship . . . and chronic human loneliness are significant contributors to premature death. . . . Almost every cause of death is significantly influenced by human companionship. Cancer . . . is significantly influenced by human companionship. . . . Nature uses many weapons to shorten the lives of lonely people.

Those are the conclusions of James J. Lynch, a physician who devoted a substantial portion of his career to studying the effect unwanted aloneness has on physical well-being. In his book *The Broken Heart: The Medical Consequences of Loneliness*, Dr. Lynch reported on one of his studies by comparing the life expectancy of the people of Nevada—who have the shortest life spans in the United States—with that of the people of Utah, who have the nation's longest life expectancy. These adjacent states are quite similar in terms of education, affluence, health consciousness, and physicians per capita.

In other respects the differences between the two states are profound. Unlike many people in Nevada, most people in Utah are religious and neither drink nor smoke. They generally maintain very stable lives. Their marriages are generally secure, family ties remain strong, and most of the state's inhabitants stay in Utah for most of their lives. Dr. Lynch concluded from that comparison that people in Utah live longer because they have deeper and longer-lasting relationships—that stable relationships promote health and prolong life.

A pamphlet published by the state of California entitled "Friends Can Be Good Medicine" proclaims: "Friends and other supportive relationships . . . are as important to your *physical well-being* as they are to your *emotional health*." The pamphlet adds that "research has shown that there is a correlation between the quality of our relationships and our physical well-being."

Two studies—the Alameda Study, conducted by Lisa F. Berkman, Ph.D., of Yale University and Lester Breslow, M.D., M.P.H., of UCLA; and the various studies of acculturated Japanese carried out by S. Leonard Syme, Ph.D., and his associates—have also clearly shown that having many social contacts has a beneficial effect on physical well-being.

The Alameda Study took a random sample of some seven thousand adults in that California county and divided them into age brackets (thirty to forty-nine, fifty to fifty-nine, and sixty to sixty-nine) and levels of social connections. No other criteria— such as weight or smoking and drinking habits—were considered. For the next nine years, the mortality of this group was monitored. In analyzing their statistics, the researchers reached a remarkable conclusion: for the people studied *the more social contacts the longer the life; the fewer the contacts the shorter the life.*

For example, the study found that in the fifty- to fifty-nine-year-old range, for every man with the most social contacts who died during the nine-year study, 3.2 men with the least social contacts died. For every socially active woman between the ages of thirty and forty-nine who died, 4.6 socially inactive women died.

The Japanese studies by Dr. Syme also found that close, continuing social contacts have a beneficial effect on health. He compared Japanese men who had come to the United States and adopted our customs to Japanese men who had remained in Japan or who had come to the U.S. mainland or Hawaii but adhered to their own family-oriented customs. The study found that the group who adopted our custom of greater social isolation suffered heart disease almost three to five times more frequently than did the group who maintained the social ties they had in Japan. Discussing this phenomenon, Dr. Syme wrote: "The maintenance of close social ties is of paramount value in Japanese culture, as is exemplified by the . . . saying that 'a rolling stone gathers no moss.' In the United States, that saying is meant to convey the idea that a person 'on the move' is more highly valued than a person 'stuck in a rut.' In Japan, moss is a highly treasured plant and the only way a stone can acquire moss (value) is to remain in the same place."

The point made by those studies is that having friends and family around us can insulate us from illness. If many and close social contacts are conducive to a long and healthy life for a well person, they are indispensable to you as a cancer patient. In cancer, friendship is good and unwanted aloneness is bad. Let's see how to stimulate the former and minimize the latter.

HOW TO AVOID UNWANTED ALONENESS

Unwanted aloneness of cancer patients can be the result of the *reclusiveness* of the patient or the *abandonment* of the patient by his or her friends and relations. I will discuss methods to overcome the abandonment of cancer patients by their friends in the next chapter and the tendency of some cancer patients to become reclusive in this chapter.

Before suggesting actions you might consider, I will review the usual reasons cancer patients become reclusive.

- They remember that before their diagnosis, it was difficult for them to be with people with cancer, and they "know" that now their well friends find it equally threatening and unpleasant to be with them.
- They are frustrated and annoyed that well people don't understand either the emotional or the physical problems they are having.

- They believe they frighten well people because well people believe that people with cancer are "doomed."
- Conversation is difficult because the cancer patient doesn't know how much others want to hear about the illness, and those others are not sure how much the cancer patient wants to tell.
- They believe that because they are wearing a colostomy bag, are bald from chemotherapy, or are pale and weak, they are so unattractive that others don't want to be with them.
- They believe that no one would want to be intimate or affectionate with a cancer patient.

Do any of these reasons sound familiar to you? Once again, this problem may not apply to you. If it doesn't, go to another chapter. If it does, read on.

When the reasons for reclusiveness are looked at objectively, it becomes apparent that they are based on the myths about cancer. That doesn't make them easy to overcome, but it can be done.

ACTIONS YOU CAN TAKE TO OVERCOME RECLUSIVENESS

STEP ONE:
Do some self-analysis to learn why you now find it more difficult to be with people than you did before the diagnosis. The most difficult part of this exercise will be to be realistic but not too hard on yourself. Start by asking yourself the following questions:

- Are you staying away from the people who were your family and friends because you believe that they don't want to be with you now?
- Do you believe that the people who loved you and enjoyed being with you before the diagnosis don't want to be with

you now? Be very clear here; this question is not about the other people. It's about you—what you believe.

- Do you believe that your friends and relations are so shallow as to leave at the first sign of adversity?
- Are you ashamed of the way you look and act because of the illness?
- If the situation were reversed, would you be so upset at their infirmity or physical condition that you would shun them? If your answer is no, why do you believe your friends and family are so much less understanding than you are? Why do you believe that their love and affection is based only on trouble-free times?

Don't sell your friends and family short. Assume that they want to continue to be part of your life, and understand that if they are acting strangely, it's because of their fear or lack of knowledge about the illness. Also examine whether your demands on their loyalty and love are reasonable under the circumstances. Remember that they have lives independent of yours.

STEP TWO:
Ask yourself and your friends how you have changed since the diagnosis. Is your attitude with your friends and family much as it was before the illness, or is it that of consummate victim?

The first set of questions is designed to help you consider your state of mind about companionship. This latter question will help you analyze your conduct so that you can make such adjustments as you believe to be in your best interest.

Then, with all of this self-knowledge, and with the understanding that your level of activity may be curtailed by physical problems, the advice is—don't be more reclusive than your physical condition requires and take part in as many interactions with friends and relations as you can. Do it as part of your fight for recovery. One of the happy parts of involving yourself in the fight for recovery at this level is that it doesn't have the unpleasant side effects of chemotherapy, radiation, and surgery.

CHAPTER 16

Don't Let Your Family and Friends Abandon You

Sometimes families and friends unconsciously abandon people with cancer. Abandonment, and that word is more dramatic than necessary but the only one that seems to work, can be physical, where your friends actually stay away from you, or emotional, where their reaction to cancer makes conversation so stilted and sterile that they might as well have stayed away. In this chapter I will discuss actions you can take to counter this not unusual reaction, and counter it you should, because unwanted aloneness is an unpleasant emotion that depresses the immune system.

If you experienced a significant change in your relationships after your diagnosis—if it appears to you that your friends and relations are now not as close to you as they were—all my experience indicates that you can be sure it's not because they love you less. It's simply that most well people are uncomfortable being with people with cancer—even those they love. Possibly you had the same reaction to cancer patients before your diagnosis. Such reflex action of withdrawal has been well documented. Camille Wortman, Ph.D., a noted psychologist who has done extensive work in this field, wrote: "In [one] study of the perceived support available to breast cancer patients, seventy-two percent of the respondents reported that they were treated differently after people knew they had cancer. Of these, seventy-five percent indicated that they were misunderstood by others and over fifty percent reported that they were 'avoided' or 'feared.' "

Susan Sontag, in her book *Illness as Metaphor,* wrote: "A surprisingly large number of people with cancer find themselves being shunned by relatives and friends and are the object of practices of decontamination by members of their household, as if cancer, like tuberculosis, were an infectious disease. Contact with someone afflicted with the disease regarded as a mysterious malevolency feels [to them] like a trespass."

And L. M. Videka, in a report entitled "Psychosocial Adaptations in a Medical Self-Help Group," wrote: "This general high need of ill people for increased social support comes at a time when those supports are seriously diminished. For example, people with serious illness (especially cancer) are often faced with isolation from friends and family because of fear of contagion, fear of expression of intense emotions or because [the others] don't wish to be reminded of their own vulnerability."

The experience of many Wellness Community participants supports these viewpoints. We have all watched cancer patients becoming more and more isolated simply because they have cancer. But quite probably, you don't need this book or any scientific literature to tell you about cancer-induced aloneness. Unless you have an unusual family and friends, isolation is probably part of your own experience. Family and friends distance themselves from cancer patients for a number of reasons:

- They can't bear to be with someone they know and love when they feel this person is suffering and ultimately doomed. They believe the myths also.
- Being with the cancer patient makes them acutely aware of their own vulnerability and their own mortality.
- The only subject they can think about when they are with the person with cancer is the illness, and yet they are determined that the word "cancer" shall never pass their lips in the presence of the cancer patient.
- They feel inadequate because they want to help and there is nothing they can do.
- They are afraid that cancer is contagious.

- They are afraid the cancer patient will tell them the truth about how he or she feels, and they are sure that they won't be able to bear it.

I am reminded of a statement made by a Wellness Community participant when discussing this subject: "When they ask you how you are, and you answer, 'Okay,' that's the end of that conversation. They really don't want to know. To people who love you, actually knowing how you feel would be devastating."

Some of the suggestions in this chapter can help put your friends and family at ease so that you can resume life together and have their support in your fight for recovery.

ACTIONS YOU CAN TAKE TO HELP YOUR FAMILY CONTINUE TO INTERACT WITH YOU AS THEY DID BEFORE

STEP ONE:

Talk to your friends and family directly and openly about this subject:

Ask for their help. Tell them you want the relationship to go on as it was before. Do you see what I just did? I suggested that you ask for help. When this type of suggestion is made, very often the reaction is: "Horrors! What did you say— ask for help? Not me. I'll never ask for help. I never have and I never will." The underlying discomfort that prompts this response is based on the unasked question "What if I ask for their help and they turn me down? I will be mortified." Perhaps you recognize this less than realistic or adult, but completely understandable, reaction.

But let me assure you that the reaction you anticipate is far worse than the reaction you will get. In all likelihood, friends and family are anxious to help. They don't want to abandon you. They just don't know how to act and they are frightened.

Betty, a forty-five-year-old widow with ovarian cancer had

two sons, twenty and twenty-two, both of whom lived with her. When the seriousness of Betty's illness became apparent, her relationship with her sons changed drastically. They stopped discussing with her all the subjects uppermost in the minds of boys in college, and they no longer brought their friends home. Although Betty's friends made sure she was never alone, they would not talk to her about the illness or their lives as they did before. Betty recalled:

> One day, my sons and I began having the same dumb conversations. And I became furious. I yelled and screamed. I told them they were treating me as if I weren't there, and that this was depressing me. I told them that I was still a part of their lives and they were still a part of mine and that I wanted to be treated that way. It wasn't a conversation; it was a screaming match. We then all began to laugh and cry, the dam overflowed—and everything changed. They still treat me as if I am sick, because I am. But once again, I am their mother and they are my sons. I know they love me and want to help me.
>
> After that, it was easy to tell my friends what I thought of the way they were treating me. Some of them understood immediately and changed; some of them just couldn't. But my life is now back to where I look forward to being with people.

Telling your friends and family what you want from them is really all you can do. You can't change anyone but yourself. However, if those close to you don't adopt your suggestions immediately, you don't have to let that be the end of the relationship. Keep trying. Don't forget that for most of them, this is a new experience and resuming the relationship as it was before can be difficult. When you ask for their help you are breaking what is probably a lifelong pattern for both you and them. Most people have never had anybody speak to them candidly and openly about their wants and desires. Many of them have never experienced or contemplated shared intimacy and real, unreserved friendship. In most cases, you are asking them to consciously act in a way they have never acted before. So don't be surprised if it takes them some time to respond in the way you want them to.

STEP TWO:
Ask yourself and your friends how you have changed since the diagnosis. Maybe there's a reason they seem to be staying away from you. There is the possibility that you have changed some aspect of your behavior which makes being with you more difficult than it was before. If they are staying away, you might ask yourself questions like some of the following:

- Have I become too demanding?
- Is the illness my only topic of conversation?
- Am I taking advantage of the situation so that others are required to perform tasks that actually are my responsibility?
- Am I forcing others to allow me to act in ways that would otherwise be unacceptable?
- Is my attitude with my friends and family much as it was before the illness, or is it that of consummate victim?

These are questions worthy of careful consideration. So stop now, and reread and think about them. Just understanding the issues, even without fully knowing the answers, can affect the quality of your life, and therefore perhaps the course of the illness.

A warning: When you ask for other people's opinions, listen to what they say, but decide for yourself what's best for you. Don't be surprised if some people fail you; they have problems of their own—fear of facing their own mortality, for example. And some of them just can't make the change. Different circumstances spawn different friends. And your circumstances have certainly changed. It's quite possible that your circle of friends will, too.

I have a large family—four brothers and four sisters and many nieces and nephews. Even though we were scattered all over the United States, we were all close until about five years ago. It was then an argument started at a family affair. It wasn't a major argument but everyone got caught up in it and somehow after that, we all stopped talking to each other. I wasn't happy about it—but somehow I didn't do anything about it either. About two years ago I was diagnosed with lymphoma and I realized I might die. Without a second thought, my new wife, who had never met any of the family, and I planned a party for all of my relatives. We called them all and everyone that could came to our party. There were over forty people there. We cried and laughed and told each other how dumb we were to have let so much time pass. That was about six months ago and was one of the smartest things I've ever done. My phone bills are high, but so are my spirits.

Leo

CHAPTER 17

Seek Family Harmony

Cancer always has a profound effect on the entire family. This effect can be positive, making the members more aware of how much they mean to each other, or it can place intolerable pressure on the relationships. It is my experience that the possibility of the latter taking place is much less likely if the people involved clearly communicate their wants and needs. Unfortunately, this happens all too seldom because in most families the members communicate their needs not by the spoken word but by body language and facial expressions; that leaves everybody guessing and very often they guess wrong. Perhaps you recognize that type of family.

"If we love each other, we should know how the other feels without having to express it." That was the statement made by the husband of a cancer patient, interviewed as part of a study by A. Koch, Ph.D. He couldn't have been more wrong. No matter how long a couple or a family has lived together, no one really knows what the other is thinking or feeling unless and until he or she is told.

Jimmie C. Holland, M.D., a noted authority on this subject, observed the following in a 1982 interview: "Family members are under enormous stress—sometimes as great as that of the cancer patient himself. Members of the family often have the same feelings of hopelessness/helplessness, passivity, anger, anxiety, and all of the other negative emotions experienced by the cancer patient."

And the stress is filled with confusing and contradictory emotions. Cancer patients becomes angry and frustrated when their families treat them as they did before the illness: "Don't they know how sick I am?" Or they become just as angry if they are treated as an invalid. They grow distant because they can't tell their families how frightened they are: "If they knew, they couldn't handle it." And they pull away because they can't interact as they once did. The cancer patient worries about the strain he or she is placing on the family, both financial and emotional, and the rest of the family, worrying about the identical issues, feel guilty that they are not being as loyal as they should be. So no matter what reaction your family is experiencing, it is not abnormal—you and your family are just like the rest of us. That takes care of one worry.

These unpleasant and immune-depressing conditions can be minimized by open and direct communication. Troublesome emotions become much less ominous when they are shared, and that means talking about them. So the basic rule to help ease the strain on the family brought about by cancer and in many other situations is: Communicate, communicate, communicate. Tell them what you want and need and how you would like them to change. Ask them how they would like you to change. You love each other—try it.

One family (mother with cancer, father, sons sixteen and eighteen, and daughter eleven) devised its own approach to opening up communication. At least one night each week after dinner, everyone who was home would sit together for a short time and discuss their feelings. Sometimes it grew heavy and there were tears, but they reported that it was always worth it. One aspect they insisted on was that each was to tell some happy or worthwhile event that had happened that week. This simple device, they said, kept the family together. It sounds like a good idea to me— particularly the part about telling at least one happy story at each meeting. It seems to me that those happy stories will make everyone aware that life is more than just cancer, and that joy and pleasure in some form and in some quantity are still there for the taking.

But you don't need a formal arrangement. You just have to

talk openly and candidly with each other. Once again, don't hear me saying that this is an easy task. It isn't. We are not used to talking to each other about ourselves and our emotions. But it's a skill that can be learned and improved by practice and can solve a great many problems. I suggest you try it.

I had two brain operations before I came to a meeting at The Wellness Community on the topic of "The Family and Cancer." There were about twenty-five other cancer patients and their families there. I was twenty-nine and my mother, father, and sister came with me. We all lived together. During that meeting, I started to talk about the second operation and how terribly afraid I was that the cancer would reappear, and I started to cry. I hadn't talked about my fear with my family because I didn't want them to be frightened too. When my mother saw my tears, she took me in her arms as she did when I was a very little girl, and we sat there crying together. My father and sister moved closer and we all held hands. They told me later that they didn't want to intrude. My mother, still holding me tight, said she had always known about my fear because the entire family were worried about the same thing but that they didn't want me to worry about them. So now it was out in the open. We loved each other and we were all too frightened to talk to each other and now we could talk about anything.

Michelle

NOTE: I happened to be in the room when this took place and I can tell you that the release and relief they felt was apparent not only on their faces but on the faces of the other twenty-five people in the room.

CHAPTER 18

◁‒

Spend Time with Other Cancer Patients

In the previous chapters I suggested spending time with your friends and family, because being with friends and family dispels unwanted aloneness. The suggestion made here is that you also spend some time with other cancer patients, because being with other cancer patients who understand exactly what you are going through not only avoids aloneness but also provides a feeling of belonging which somehow was lost with the diagnosis. I will suggest how you can meet other cancer patients at the end of this chapter.

Many Wellness Community participants have told me they believe that the relationships with other cancer patients have been a major benefit of The Wellness Community program and an integral part of their fight for recovery. They say that it is impossible for any well person to appreciate the always nagging fear and lack of control that impinge upon every area of life, and the way the illness makes it difficult to make even the simplest plans. These same people tell me, "We cancer patients share an enormous number of experiences unknown to all but the initiated, and those shared experiences foster a calmness that is difficult if not impossible to achieve with well persons."

Don't expect to bond with every cancer patient you meet but it's quite likely that you will receive some benefit from even those who aren't exactly your type.

To be able to describe just how important cancer patients

believe it is to be with other cancer patients, I attended a Wellness Community orientation meeting—the meeting where cancer patients first learn how The Wellness Community can help them. Those meetings are led by cancer patients who are familiar with The Wellness Community and who have recovered or are doing well with the illness. In the room the night I was there were seventeen people new to The Wellness Community, and Wellness Community participants Greg, a twenty-six-year-old patient who had been fighting bladder cancer for several years and had been asymptomatic for quite a while, and Doris, who had been fighting colon cancer for over a year. The benefits of being with other cancer patients was discussed first by Greg, who said: "When I heard the diagnosis, I immediately knew that I didn't belong in the same world with those who were well. I had become different. Meeting and being with other cancer patients who had gone through what I was going through restored my feelings of oneness with my universe. They understand me and I understand them. They didn't give me pity, they give me understanding."

Doris described her experience as follows: "Until recently I always felt a great deal of strain being with my well friends. I found myself constantly shielding them from my real fears and pain so that they wouldn't be upset. Or I was fighting back my annoyance because they didn't understand the seriousness of my illness, or I was irked by the fact that they were not relating to me in the same way they did before. And sometimes I was resentful and jealous because they were well and I was ill, and at other times I thought they felt superior to me for the same reason. As you can see, those reactions weren't rational, but there they were. With other cancer patients, on the other hand, I am relaxed. They understand."

Greg then drew an interesting analogy. He proposed that there was a great similarity between cancer patients and people who are part of a disaster like a flood or a hurricane. He based his analogy on an article that described a study performed by UCLA researcher Linda Nelson, Ph.D. After studying people involved in more than twenty natural disasters over the past sixty years, Dr. Nelson concluded, "Residents in the stricken communities generally keep their heads, care for one another, share common resources, and *actually reach an emotional high as they pull together and tackle the common challenges of survival and rebuilding.* Many of them," she added, "feel saddened at some level when the crisis is over; they realize that they have never experienced that emotion before and perhaps never will again." Greg then observed that cancer patients also face an enormous challenge and benefit in exactly the same way by being together and sharing the trials and tribulations they are all going through. He said, "I know the emotional high Dr. Nelson is talking about. I've been there."

Some cancer patients describe the benefit they receive from being with other patients in terms of an esprit de corps. They recognize that they are experiencing the same warmth of togetherness so prevalent in groups of people who have joined together to fight a common enemy—such as soldiers, firefighters, and police officers.

The basic emotion expressed by many cancer patients is summed up in this statement: "I want to be with you because you understand, because we are sharing a crisis, because no matter that we have just met, you recognize in me what I see in you, and because of that your well-being is important to me and I know that you want the best for me and care what happens to me. I don't have to explain to you or hide from you either the fears or the hopes for the future that lie deep inside me, because I know that you are feeling those same fears and hopes."

One study, published in 1983 by the Rand Corporation, called "Measuring the Ability to Cope with Serious Illness" also deals with the possibility that cancer patients benefit from being with other cancer patients. Its author, Anita Stewart, Ph.D., writes: "It has been suggested that seriously ill people have a particular need for support from other seriously ill patients—from others who have experienced the same problems and feelings." And she points out that "people cope more effectively with disability when they have a firm sense of belonging in a highly valued group such as a family or community."

There is one more issue to be addressed here: the reluctance of some cancer patients to become friends with others with cancer for fear of the emotional trauma if the newfound friend does not do as well as hoped. Although this is a reasonable cause for misgivings, the relevant question here is: "Shall I forgo the possible benefits and pleasures of a new friend who has cancer—and who therefore understands me better than anyone else can—because of the possibility that the relationship will end sooner than I want it to?"

Gilda Radner in her book *It's Always Something* answers that question. She says, "The hardest part of committing myself to The Wellness Community and becoming friends with people was learning later that someone who had become close had died. The course of cancer isn't always what we hope. I was learning that death is a part of life. But if I hadn't gone to The Wellness Community, think of all the love I would have missed. While we have the gift of life, it seems to me the only tragedy is to allow a part of us to die—whether it is our spirit, our creativity or our glorious uniqueness."

All Wellness Community participants have opted in favor of friendship. They have integrated into their psyche the concept that under all circumstances—sick or well—one has no alternative but to accept the eventuality of the death of a friend, and that it is in their best interest to appreciate the joy of the present with full knowledge of how tenuous the future is. Most Wellness Community participants would recommend that you take the chance and, through me, they assure you that the odds are good that you will experience the same benefit from being with other cancer patients as they did.

If you want to give it a try, you can find other cancer patients wherever you are. Ask your doctor or the nurses you interact with or the people at the hospital, or call the American Cancer Society or a Wellness Community in your area. Look up a hot line in the Yellow Pages under "Cancer." In all but the most remote regions of the country, there are organizations that will help you find other cancer patients. Remember, you probably won't like every other cancer patient you meet, but wouldn't it be wonderful if you met at least one with whom you can interact in this very special way.

CHAPTER 19

〜

Join a Support Group

As discussed in the previous chapter, there can be significant benefit to interacting with other cancer patients. In this chapter I am suggesting that, as a part of your fight for recovery, you be with other cancer patients in a very special way—in a cancer-patient support group. Being with other cancer patients in such a group enhances and augments the benefits of interacting with them by providing a forum conducive to intimate sharing and a deeper bonding. This can be important since, I believe, the closer the relationship the more immune-enhancing it will be.

I know, from being involved with groups since 1982, that groupmates become extended family—that is, they treat you as a friend with cancer rather than as a doomed object of pity; they are not so threatened by the possible eventual outcome of the illness (as are most family members) that all conversations are stilted and awkward; they do not react to your day-to-day problems with resentment; and your discomfort is not so devastating to them as to make social intercourse impossible.

The significance of this extended family cannot be over-emphasized. As we know, unwanted aloneness is one of the most crippling psychosocial impediments to the cancer patient's recovery. And one of the ideal means of warding off the ill effects of unwanted aloneness is a support group.

A cancer support group is usually a group of twelve cancer

patients who meet weekly, led by licensed psychotherapists. In The Wellness Community, our groups are called Participant Groups and our specially trained therapists are called facilitators. Facilitators, although well trained and experienced, are not the authorities in a Wellness Community Participant Group—the participants are. The facilitators facilitate interaction among the participants.

From the day The Wellness Community opened, support groups were an integral part of the program, and the fundamental principle on which the entire program was based was summed up in the following statement: "If you participate in your fight for recovery along with your physician and other health care professionals, you will probably improve the quality of your life and *may* enhance the possibility of your recovery." Notice the two benefits of acting as a Patient Active—(1) improvement of the quality of life and (2) perhaps an improved possibility of recovery. That those benefits are probably available through participating in a support group has now, some ten years later, been confirmed by two impressive recent studies.

The first study was conducted by David Spiegel, M.D., and his associates at Stanford University School of Medicine, started in 1985 and ended in 1993. In the study fifty women with metastatic breast cancer joined weekly support groups for one year. The original purpose of the study was to determine the effect that participation in such a group had on the women's quality of life. Thirty-six women with the same illness served as controls—they were not in groups and received no psychological assistance. All the women maintained routine oncological care. Immediately after the completion of the year of groups in 1986, Dr. Spiegel commented on the results of his study as follows:

. . . Support groups can clearly improve the quality of life. We were able to show reduced mood disturbances. Patients were also less phobic, they had better coping responses, and they had reduced pain. In a psychosocial sense, groups work, and a number of studies illustrate this . . .

Eight years later Dr. Spiegel examined the records of the participants in the study to determine whether or not their participation in the groups had any effect on the extension of life. He found that those women who participated in the support groups lived twice as long as those who did not. However, Dr. Spiegel warns us:

. . . This effect [improved quality of life and extended survival time], if it's there, comes not by denying the illness or wishing it away, but by more successfully managing one's life in terms of family relationships, relationships with physicians . . . and dealing with these factors as directly as possible.

A good reason for working hard in a group once you are in one is Dr. Spiegel's finding that there is a reasonable possibility that the degree of participation will affect the results—that is, that the more you attend the more positive the results. He said:

These figures [which showed that the women who came to the group most often survived the longest] indicate that there was something of a dose response among those randomized to treatment which suggests that something about being in a [support] group was relevant to their survival time.

The second study was conducted by Fawzy I. Fawzy, M.D., and associates at UCLA in 1989. The study was designed to evaluate the immediate and long-term effects that a six-week program of weekly group support would have on the quality of life of malignant melanoma patients. The groups focused on health education, stress management (e.g., relaxation techniques), enhancement of problem-solving skills, and psychological support. Sixty-eight Stage I and II melanoma patients who had already been operated on were randomly assigned to either the group intervention or a control condition. There were thirty-four in each group. All patients received standard medical and surgical treatment. The patients in the control group did not participate in support groups or any other psychiatric intervention.

The study was in two stages. Immediately after the completion of the study, Dr. Fawzy commented on the effect groups have on quality of life as follows:

Few dispute the reported beneficial effects [of psychosocial group intervention] in relation to improvements in affective distress, coping behavior, quality of life, and pain control. At the end of the psychiatric intervention [groups], the intervention patients [those who were in the groups] exhibited significantly lower levels of distress and greater use of positive coping methods than the controls. At six months follow-up, the group differences were even more pronounced. The intervention group patients showed significantly lower depression, fatigue, confusion and total mood disturbance as well as higher vigor. They were also using significantly more active-behavioral and active-cognitive coping than the controls. At the one year follow-up, the intervention group continued to show significantly lower confusion and higher vigor.

Then, five years later, Dr. Fawzy and his colleagues analyzed the longevity of the participants in the study. Their findings led Dr. Fawzy to make the following statement in relation to the extension of life:

Psychiatric interventions [support groups] that are aimed at enhancing effective coping and reduction of distress seem to have a beneficial effect on survival.

Certainly, these studies are not the final word on the effect that groups have on survival, but they are a most encouraging first step.

HISTORY

That group therapy can be an effective tool in the Patient Active's fight for recovery is not a new concept. Chronically ill people participated in such groups as early as the turn of the century, and their popularity burgeoned in the 1970s. At a 1976 American Cancer Society conference on group counseling with cancer patients and their families, Irving Yalom, M.D., of the Stanford Medical School ended his address by saying:

> Some of the [cancer] patients who have worked most effectively in a group have come very far. What we've seen is that the confrontation [with a life-threatening illness in the group] for many people has resulted in a richer mode of living . . . than was true for them before their cancer. They are able to trivialize the trivia in their lives and alter their life perspective—not to do things they really don't want to do. . . . It's kind of a liberating feeling involving more willingness to take risks . . . and perhaps setting certain goals.

Then in 1980, in her American Psychological Association presidential address, Leona Tyler, M.D., who had done extensive research in this field, suggested that by the year 2000, support groups will be the primary vehicle for dealing with health-related psychosocial issues.

How important can these groups be? In Jane Goldberg's book *Psychotherapeutic Treatment of Cancer Patients,* N. Miller, M.D., an authority on the subject, is quoted thus: "Limiting the treatment [of cancer] to medical remedies only is analogous to trying to save a sinking ship by bailing out the water while ignoring the holes in the bottom of the ship."

Almost all Wellness Community participants join and participate regularly in cancer-patient support groups. We call them Participant Groups. One of them was Kari, a freelance writer in her mid-forties. Kari had had an adenocarcinoma surgi-

cally removed from her left lung about six months before making the following statement:

> I became part of a participant group because I was terrified,
> and I didn't want to be alone. I wanted to be with people
> who were experiencing the same aftereffects of cancer I was.
> I knew that cancer had changed my life both physically and
> mentally forever, and I felt, and I still feel, a very strong need
> to be around people to whom I can talk, so that I don't feel
> alone. And when I'm scared, I know that there is someone
> who will listen to me and not be frightened by what I'm
> saying.
>
> If my mother asks me how I am, the question is so loaded
> with emotional overtones that a straight answer is almost
> impossible. If my friend becomes angry with me, she's afraid to
> show it—she's afraid of me since I became ill. But in my
> group, everybody is in the same boat and has experienced the
> same problems I have. I don't frighten them.
>
> From the group, we all receive the courage to keep trying.
> When you feel sick and vulnerable, it's very hard to keep
> going, to try to change things and take control. Without a
> group, I don't know how people "get it together" to say, "I
> want this treatment," when Dr. A says one thing and Dr. B
> another, and your instincts tell you a third.
>
> One of the most important results of my participation in
> the group is that the group became the catalyst for learning the
> lessons cancer had to teach. If I'm depressed about something
> unrelated to cancer, I can bring it to my group. And by hearing
> how others would handle the same situation, I learn new
> methods of attacking problems, and I can get rid of the stress in
> my life.
>
> I have also learned many skills in my group that I can use
> the rest of my life. For instance, I have learned to talk to myself.
> When I face a problem, I consciously discuss the various
> possibilities with myself and with others. That helps a lot in
> making the right decision.

Not only is it healthy to have many social contacts, but there is the reasonable hypothesis that the deeper, the more meaningful, and the longer-lasting the friendships are, the greater effect they will have on your immune system. And there is no better way to build such relationships than to be with other people with cancer in a support group in which you expose your weaknesses and foibles and ask for help, and in which others do the same with you.

Caution: Not every group is a good group, so when deciding whether to join a group I would suggest you follow these guidelines:

- Be sure that it is in support of conventional medical treatment.
- Discuss participation with your physician or some physician who is familiar with the work of the group.
- Leave quickly any group that tells you
  1. that you should give up conventional medical treatment,
  2. that you are at fault for the onset of the illness,
  3. that you are solely responsible for the course of the illness.
- Leave quickly any group
  1. where they give you instructions rather than observations,
  2. where they have all the answers,
  3. where everybody is always gloomy and depressed.

HOW TO ACT IN A SUPPORT GROUP

Once you become part of a group, or decide to be open with your cancer friend or friends as a part of your fight for recovery, treat the experience as an important part of your total effort. Get down to essentials as soon as possible—that is, talk about yourself. Reveal as much about yourself as you can. Tell them about matters you have never discussed before. You probably will fib and shade the truth in the beginning; everybody does. But be as honest and open as you can. You are doing it *for you*. The faster you find out what parts of your life you are hiding—which are therefore stress-producing—the sooner you can do something about them.

If you can't find a support group, you might also consider private therapy if you can afford it, or look for a facility where you can receive counseling without charge. But be sure that any therapist you use understands what you are looking for and knows that you are in therapy because you believe or hope it will help your recovery process. While private therapy can't give you the social contacts or the extended family you need, it can help you find areas of stress in your life. However, if the therapist wants to teach you to take a resigned, passive stance vis-à-vis your diagnosis and prognosis—and that's all he or she wants to do—that therapist is not for you. You want to be a Patient Active. You want to fight for your recovery.

To find a support group, call the American Cancer Society (1-800-4-CANCER), or write or call The Wellness Community nearest you or the national organization in Santa Monica, California (310-314-2555), or Make Today Count, 1235 East Cherokee, Springfield, MO 65804 (1-800-432-2273), or Cancer Care Inc., 1180 Avenue of the Americas, New York, NY 10036 (212-221-3300). To locate other cancer patients, ask your doctor for some names or call a cancer hot line. A listing of additional resources appears in Appendix 6.

IS PARTICIPATING IN GROUPS OR BEING WITH OTHER CANCER PATIENTS TOO DEPRESSING?

Some cancer patients are concerned that they might find being in a group or with other cancer patients too depressing. This concern is valid up to a point. The social interaction with other cancer patients that is inspiring for some is found by others to be so depressing that continued participation is not in their best interest. In truth, support programs are not for everyone. However, experience at The Wellness Community since 1982 indicates that those who find the interaction with other cancer patients too depressing leave after the first session without harm being done. On the other hand, the cancer patients who do participate in support programs on an ongoing basis accommodate to the possibility of death and revel in the fact that they had each other during the fight for recovery. The decision is yours.

CHAPTER 20

◦⌒⌒

Form a Partnership with Your Physicians

"During recent years there has been a marked change in the way people in our society, including health experts, view the role of the patient." That is the opinion of Irving L. Janis of Yale University as expounded in the book *Handbook of Behavioral Medicine*. He goes on to say: "No longer are patients seen as passive recipients of health care who are expected to do willingly whatever the doctor says. Rather, they are increasingly regarded as active decision makers, making crucial choices that can markedly affect the kind of treatment they receive and the outcome."

That new relationship is what this chapter is about, because your relationship with your doctor is of extreme importance to you. A good relationship with a person you are going to interact with on a fairly consistent basis over a period of time, and who plays such an important part in your life, certainly makes life more pleasant. More important, it is thought by many professionals that the quality of the relationship may have some effect on the efficacy of the treatment. The theory is that although medicine administered by a physician you do not respect or trust will probably have the physiological effect for which it is designed, it probably won't have the same curative power as the identical medicine administered by a physician in whom you have complete confidence. Herbert Benson, M.D., underscored the importance of the patient-physician relationship when he wrote that the placebo effect (the body's ability to heal itself) works when three elements are present: "one, the belief and expectation of the patient; two, the belief and expectation of the physician; and three, *the interaction between the patient and the physician.*"

Thus, the quality of the interaction between you and your physician is not a matter to be left to chance. But a rocky beginning for this relationship is not uncommon, because the cancer patient's first reaction after diagnosis is often shock and disbelief, followed by the "Why me?" syndrome and then unreasoning anger. At that time, what the patient wants to hear more than anything else is that the diagnosis is a mistake, or at least that the illness will be of brief duration and leave no lasting effects. And who but the physician is the one who must disappoint the patient in this regard, while prescribing medications, procedures, and tests that can have unpleasant side effects. As a result, it's not unusual for the patient's anger to land on the physician, setting up a delicate and sometimes uncomfortable situation.

Although a great majority of physicians respond as caring fellow human beings, there are a few who do eliminate all hope, who are distant, who won't answer questions, and who treat the patient like a not too bright employee. Even when the physician is sensitive and caring, a doctor-patient dance always ensues, with the physician doing the leading.

In the early stages of the illness, all of the responsibility falls upon the physician, who is at no risk, is the professional, and has been in similar circumstances many times before. The doctor should be, and the great majority are, prepared for the reactions of the patient, and should have developed some way to transmit information to a frightened, bewildered person in a manner that is supportive, hopeful, positive, yet accurate.

Of course, a medical degree does not bestow sainthood or unlimited patience, and a physician cannot be expected to act forever as a caring friend and confidant to an overly demanding, hostile, and angry patient. As in every interaction, the patient-physician connection must be a two-way street.

In many respects, the patient-physician relationship is the same as a business relationship with any independent contractor, such as a lawyer, accountant, plumber, or mechanic; each is paid for doing the best he or she can to accomplish the desired results. But physicians are special in several ways. They help us maintain or regain our most precious possession, our health. In no other situation does the independent contractor have so much responsibility. In no other situation is it quite so important that his or her advice and ministrations be correct, and that errors of both judgment and performance be avoided. In few other situations is so much training required and are so many obligations placed on the independent contractor.

One of those obligations is to instill confidence and a feeling of security in the patient, while not appearing too authoritarian or remote. This is a difficult role to play, and woe to the physician who fails us in any way or does not perform as expected.

Because a good relationship with the right physician is of overriding importance to you, you should probably commit as much time and energy as is necessary to attain such a relationship. The following are steps that may be helpful:

STEP ONE:
Choose a medically competent physician. In most cases, this is done by recommendation and reputation. There are also situations where your insurance carrier or HMO will select your physician.

STEP TWO:
Ensure that the relationship is, at the very least, cordial. It does not have to blossom into a full-blown friendship for it to be effective and efficient. It is only necessary that it be agreeable. One of our participants summed up his perception of his role in this relationship as follows:

As a cancer patient, I cannot think of anyone whose approval I am more interested in than my oncologist's. I want him to think of me as a decent, reasonable man who wants to recover more than anything else in the world. While he may not look forward to the day he is scheduled to see me, I wouldn't want him to dread it.

In order to be worthy of my doctor's respect, I am, within my own capabilities, courteous, friendly, and considerate of his time. I am careful that my demands on him are reasonable. I try to be constantly aware that he is not a God who can cure me with a wave of his hand, that he has other patients, and that his entire life does not revolve around me alone.

STEP THREE:

Make sure that the expectations of both you and your doctor are clearly understood by each of you. There are as many variations of the patient-physician relationship as there are patients and doctors. Some patients want every bit of information they can get. Others want to hear nothing but instructions. Some want to know what the treatment alternatives are and want to make the final decisions themselves. Others want the doctor to decide what's best. Some consider waiting in a waiting room an acceptable inconvenience, while others find it intolerable. Some want to ask questions, write down answers, and have other people in the examining room. Other's don't. Physicians, just like everyone else, are also different and those differences must also be taken into account.

In a paper discussing the importance of a good patient-physician relationship, Howard Leventhal, Ph.D., and his colleagues at the University of Wisconsin discussed the necessity that each clearly understand the expectations of the other: "Both patient and physician have specific expectations of and preferences for the type of relationship they will enjoy and the outcome they expect from their interactions. The expectations held by each party may differ considerably; and these differences may go unrecognized. Since the relationship places the physician in general control of the interaction, the substance of the relationship is likely to conform more closely to his or her expectations. Thus, to the extent that the patient's and physician's expectations differ, the patient may ultimately be unhappy with the care and may be less likely to remain in and comply with the treatment."

Frank discussions are therefore indicated, preferably after a reasonable breaking-in period during which you have become aware of what your needs are and how your doctor is responding to them. At the first of these discussions you should probably decide with your doctor how much you want to know and what part you want to play in the decision-making process. Make sure that those issues are clear between you and that you both agree.

Very often, it is difficult for the patient to start the conversation with the doctor. After all, physicians have always been authority figures. But start it anyway. With very few exceptions, your physician is as anxious to have the conversation as you are. The dialogue should continue as long as necessary and you should probably initiate new conversations when any part of the relationship appears unsatisfactory.

STEP FOUR:

If your needs as a patient conflict seriously with the doctor's style, consider whether it's in your best interest to find another physician. Most people find it difficult and sometimes embarrassing to leave a physician. Although this rather drastic step should be taken only after serious consideration, it's not impossible or unthinkable. If the situation is irreparable, it's appropriate.

Often cancer patients are treated by a group of physicians that may include an oncologist, radiologist, surgeon, and/or some other specialist, along with the family doctor. One of the patient's most frequent complaints is that no one is in charge—each physician acts almost independently—and there is no one to whom the patient can talk to get *all* the information needed to make a decision. Therefore, it's important that you try to get one of the doctors to be the coordinator of the team and the repository of all information.

One admonition: Don't ask for a prognosis or inquire about longevity statistics unless you are actually ready to hear the answer.

Most physicians are cautious about making predictions about longevity because they just don't know what an individual's life expectancy will be. If hard-pressed, they will discuss the statistics but will also describe patients who substantially outlived the statistics or who recovered completely.

Several years ago, I had a discussion with about twenty participants to discuss their relationship with their physicians. From that dialogue, it became apparent that most of them had complete confidence in their physicians and were generally happy with their relationship. But there were also some horror stories, particularly about physicians stripping the patient of hope.

This interchange raised the question of what a cancer patient could reasonably expect from a physician. To answer those questions, I met with five oncologists on The Wellness Community's Professional Advisory Board. At that meeting, the oncologists concurred that some patients, while receiving proper medical care, had relationships with their physicians that were not the most conducive to recovery, and that many patients believed that insensitive treatment by their doctors was normal. After five meetings of this group, we prepared a statement we called "The Wellness Community Patient/Oncologist Statement" and tested it by distribution to three hundred cancer patients. It is designed to help you judge whether your relationship with your own oncologist is all it should be. A copy of that statement appears in Appendix 2.

As a prelude to writing this book, I asked another group of patients to look over that statement to see if it was still current, and I was assured that it was. You might show it to your physician and discuss it with him or her.

GUIDELINES FOR VISITS WITH PHYSICIANS

The following guidelines are designed to help you more thoroughly understand the instructions given to you, and will probably result in greater peace of mind and instill in you more confidence in your physician.

- Before the visit prepare a written list of the questions you want to ask your doctor, to ensure that all your questions are asked.
- For the same reasons, before the visit, prepare a written list of the information you want the doctor to know.
- If you don't understand something your doctor says, say so. If you don't speak up, you may follow the wrong advice or take an improper amount of medication.
- Take someone with you when you visit your doctor. Your friend will not be as stressed as you and will be able to listen to and understand the doctor with greater objectivity.
- Get a second opinion when a major course of action is contemplated.
- Decide with your physician who is to make the final decision as to the treatment or if you will make that decision together.

You should do everything in your power to ensure that your relationship with your physician is as trouble-free as possible. Make certain that any problems between you and your doctor are not your fault, and then discuss any problem areas with him. If that doesn't work, find a new physician.

COMPLY WITH THE INSTRUCTIONS OF YOUR PHYSICIAN

The suggestion that you comply with your physician's instructions is so self-evident that it is difficult to write about. The title says it all. How do you explain to an adult why he or she should not cross at a busy intersection when the light is red? You say, I guess, that you shouldn't do it because you are likely to get hit by a car. It is obvious and well accepted in medical circles that noncompliance or partial compliance can result in a lowered chance of survival. That's all there is to it. What more explanation is needed? And yet, it is estimated that only 50 percent of cancer patients adequately comply with the instructions of their physicians.

Every cancer patient knows that compliance can be difficult. Nevertheless, it might be worthwhile to ask yourself the following two questions: "Am I complying with the instructions of my doctor? If I am not—why not?"

If you decide not to comply, you should make yourself aware of the risk. That's my only admonition. Be aware of what you are doing, why you are doing it, and what the likely results of non-compliance are.

A 1993 study in this area conducted by Dr. R. I. Horowitz and associates and reported in *Archives of Internal Medicine* is interesting. In that study a group of men who had survived heart attacks were divided into two groups. The first group was given a specific drug believed to enhance survival. The second group was given a placebo. The survival rate for both groups was approximately the same. However, even in the placebo group, of those who had taken the placebo consistently (at least 80 percent of the time) 15 percent died within five years. Of those who had had taken the pills less than 80 percent of the time 28 percent died. The conclusion is that there may be a beneficial effect of just taking the pills consistently. It is speculated that each time patients comply with medical instructions, they may be affirming a sense of control over the illness. How about that?

CHAPTER 21

⌒⌒

Use the Placebo Effect
Consciously

Definition: A placebo is a substance or treatment that has no curative powers, administered by someone believed to have the knowledge to "cure" illness; it is prescribed by that "knowledge-able person" with the announced purpose of curing the patient, and despite the fact that the substance has no curative power, when he uses it the patient is relieved of the symptoms. The patient has been tricked into unconsciously instructing his body to do what is necessary to recover.

Today medical science has many medicines and procedures that have curative powers. However, that is a relatively recent development. In the not too distant past medicine men, witch doctors, and physicians had many substances and performances, but very few had curative powers. Yet many patients recovered. The question as to why those recoveries took place is answered by one word—placebo.

As psychologists J. Critelli and K. Neuman have written, "the placebo was once the mainstay of medical practice. Few remedies used by physicians had any specific effect on the disorders for which they were prescribed, yet patients nonetheless improved due to the placebo effect . . . which stimulated the patient's innate capacity for self-repair." Herbert Benson, M.D., of Harvard University called attention to the placebo effect in the *Harvard Medical School Letter* in the following language: "In the past various useless agents were believed to be effective against disease: lizard's blood, crushed spiders, putrid meat, crocodile dung, bear fat, fox lungs, eunuch fat, and moss scraped from the skull of a hanged criminal. Likewise, cupping, blistering, plastering, and leeching had their day. When *both* physician and patient believed in them, these remedies could indeed have been helpful some of the time."

In his book *Anatomy of an Illness,* Norman Cousins makes the following statement:

> An understanding of the way the placebo works may be one of the most significant developments in medicine in the 20th century. It is doubtful whether the placebo—or any drug for that matter—would get very far without a patient's robust will to live. . . . The placebo has a role to play in transforming the will to live from a hypothetical conception to a physical reality and governing force. . . . *What we see ultimately is that the placebo isn't really necessary and the mind can carry out its difficult and wondrous mission unprompted by little pills. . . . The placebo is the emissary between the will to live and the body. But the emissary is expendable.* If we can liberate ourselves from tangibles, we can connect hope and the will to live directly to the ability of the body to meet great threats and challenges. The mind can carry out its ultimate functions and powers over the body without the illusion of material intervention. [Emphasis added.]

One case history, reported by Bruno Klopfer, Ph.D., is recited in many writings about the placebo effect because it illustrates so well the power of the phenomenon. In the 1950s, the drug Krebiozen was being tested as a cure for cancer. Dr. Klopfer had it administered to one of his patients with advanced cancer. The patient, who was approaching death before the administration of the drug, made a remarkable recovery and returned to many of his normal activities. Soon thereafter, testing proved the drug to be completely without curative power, and when the patient became aware of that fact, he again became "terminally ill."

At that point (and in a time when lawsuits were less threatening than they are today), Dr. Klopfer decided to take a chance. He told the patient he had obtained a new and better formula of Krebiozen and believed this drug might effect a cure. He then injected the patient with large amounts of sterile water, a placebo. Once again, the patient made an unbelievable recovery and resumed many of his normal pursuits. But soon thereafter, the patient learned of the ruse and died.

The point here is that the patient's belief in something (although it wasn't true) stimulated his body to take the actions necessary to correct the malady. If the patient had not believed in the placebo's power, his body would not have taken those curative actions. When he lost faith in the medicine, his body stopped doing those things that protected him from the illness.

Now we know that the body can be hoodwinked into effecting some miraculous results. But the vitally important question is, can you get your body to take the actions necessary for recovery (the placebo effect) without tricking it? As yet, there is no definitive answer. But Patients Active are aware that their participation in the fight for recovery along with their physicians is a useful place to start. Making the effort, being a part of the fight for recovery— just trying—may be all that's necessary.

The credo of the Patient Active then, extrapolated from knowledge of the placebo and its effect, is: "I know that under all but the most unfortunate circumstances my brain and my body are powerful enough that they can automatically return me to health. I also know that my brain can be tricked by a placebo into using that power to effect a recovery. Even though I have cancer it is possible that my body still has sufficient power to alter the course of my illness toward health and I don't want that power to lie dormant, so I will do everything in my power to consciously energize the full force of my body's power of recovery in the hope that my efforts will have a positive effect on the course of the illness. I hope that I don't need a placebo to trick me." My advice then is—do everything in your power to increase your mind's involvement in the fight for recovery and do it even though you may be skeptical about the results of your efforts. Do it because you *hope* that your efforts will be beneficial.

Once again, it is important to say that you know what's right for you better than anyone else. No matter what you do, you are doing it the very best way it can be done for you. If your efforts don't seem to be working, that's not your fault, and if anyone says it is—they're wrong.

CHAPTER 22

How to Prepare for Surgery

You should probably prepare for an operation. That's a relatively new thought but one that has been too long in coming. We now know that if you psychologically prepare for surgery or other invasive procedure, such preparation may have positive results in terms of decreased stay in the hospital after the procedure and reduced pain. This chapter is intended to be only an introduction to the area of preparation. Your physician and nursing staff are the best source of this information.

WHY YOU SHOULD PREPARE

The study in 1983 by Anita Stewart, Ph.D., of the Rand Corporation reported under the title "Measuring the Ability to Cope with Serious Illness" resulted in the following findings:

> Some [researchers] suggest that patients who have information about the amount of discomfort to be expected from an operation or other invasive procedure are able to tolerate the discomfort more easily. [Other] researchers found that having information about the physical sensations to expect during a stressful medical procedure can reduce the distress. Another found that providing patients with information about what symptoms to expect reduced complications following a heart

attack. Surgical patients who were told about postoperative pain and what could be done about it required only one half as much postoperative narcotics.

As early as 1964 a study was conducted at Massachusetts General Hospital which found that when patients have knowledge about what can be expected they benefit in many ways. In that study ninety-seven patients scheduled for surgery were randomly assigned to two groups. One group received information as to what to expect from their anesthesiologists. The control group did not receive that type of information. The group that received the education required less pain medication, experienced a faster recovery, and were discharged from the hospital 2.7 days earlier than the patients in the control group. Subsequent studies have expanded and reinforced those findings.

PREPARATIONS YOU CAN MAKE

STEP ONE:
Learn about your illness. Read books. Talk to your physician and his or her staff and other cancer patients and ex–cancer patients. The benefit of having knowledge of the illness is that it places you in a better position to discuss with your physician the merits of one procedure as compared to another and to make choices about treatment when they are presented. However, if you do not want to know all about the operation, you are not unusual. In order to determine, in a very limited way, what most cancer patients wanted in the way of information, in 1992 I asked a group of ten participants at The Wellness Community to write me a short note answering the question "How much do you want your doctor to tell you about the illness and its treatment?" All ten answered; five of them wanted all of the information they could get, three wanted to know just enough about the alternatives and possible outcomes so that they could be a part of the decision-making process, and two wanted no information at all and wanted

the physician to make all the decisions. I believe this to be a representative sampling, so no matter how you feel about this subject, you have a lot of company.

If you do want to learn about the illness, your doctor and his staff are a rich source of information. Also, there are many books on the subject. For a general overall view of cancer and its treatment, I recommend *Everyone's Guide to Cancer Therapy,* written by Drs. M. Dollinger, E. H. Rosenbaum, and E. Krames and published in 1993 by Somerville House.

STEP TWO:
Request information as to the specifics of the procedure. As the studies seem to indicate, as far as operations are concerned, forewarned is forearmed. The following are some of the areas you might want to ask your physician and nursing team about:

1. The procedures and steps you will undergo
2. The sights and sounds you will experience
3. The amount of pain you can expect
4. The methods used to control the pain
5. The amount of time it will take to recover

Try to speak to someone who has gone through the procedure. You must be careful here that the person you speak to is not a downer. You can probably learn about someone who would be a good source of information from your physician or his or her staff.

USING PSYCHOLOGICAL METHODS
TO PREPARE FOR A MEDICAL OR
SURGICAL PROCEDURE

In conversations with a great many participants of The Wellness Community and in studying the literature about such procedures, I have formulated a set of actions you might consider to prepare yourself for the operation. These are only general guidelines; as you read them you will probably devise many that are more comfortable for you. Your medical and nursing personnel are the best source for this type of information.

- Starting at least a few days before the operation, at least once or twice a day, use some type of relaxation device, such as Directed Visualization as described in Chapter 9.
- Make your stay in the hospital as comfortable as possible. Bring with you the clothing you want and the radio or cassette player you want.
- Coordinate with your anesthesiologist the use of headphones and music, and preset the volume. Plan what you will think about as you are drifting into anesthesia. Practice a script you can say to yourself as you drift off, such as: "I will be comfortable and relaxed during this procedure and I will hear only those sounds that are comfortable and helpful to me, and my body will react in the best possible way. When the operation is over I will awake calm and serene, ready to do whatever is best to speed and facilitate my recovery process."
- Find out from your physician or other health care professional what instructions you should give to your body which will be most conducive to a successful and relatively easy operation. Then, before the operation, give those instructions to your body. Example: "Body, I want you to completely relax around the site of the operation."★

These are some recommendations. I'm not suggesting that the surgery will be fun, but I do believe it will go a lot better and easier. You will also be taking back some control.

★ Here, my suggestion is that the instruction to your body be made aloud—that is, that you go into a room where no one will think you've lost your mind because you are talking to yourself, and in a determined yet loving tone of voice tell your body what you want it to do. Actually, this type of communication with your body is probably a good idea under many circumstances.

CHAPTER 23

❧

Pain—Don't Put Up with It

Although the medical treatment of cancer pain is far beyond the scope of this book, there are a few issues so well accepted in the medical community that I will pass that information on to you by quoting statements from medical authorities. Then I will discuss the psychological interventions you might use.

The most important point of this chapter is as follows: *It is imperative that you inform your physician of the degree of pain you are encountering.* If your doctor knows your pain is more severe than can be alleviated by taking aspirin, he or she will use all available means to relieve it. As is indicated by the medical authorities quoted below, (1) there is sufficient knowledge so that almost all cancer pain can be relieved, (2) most pain can be relieved without the potential of addiction or other adverse side effects, and (3) it is imperative that pain be controlled because unrelieved, severe pain has harmful physical and psychological side effects.

You may believe that because you have cancer, you have to suffer with pain. You don't! Pain, which can be debilitating and interfere with the recovery process, can usually be eliminated by medication or procedures prescribed by your physician. That's what the experts—physicians and scientists—say.

"In approximately 90% of patients cancer pain can be controlled through relatively simple means." That is the consensus statement from the 1994 National Cancer Institute Workshop on Cancer Pain as reported in "Management of Cancer Pain," a publication of the U.S. Department of Health and Human Services. That report goes on to say that the undertreatment of pain is a serious health problem. It advises that ". . . every patient with cancer should have the expectation of pain control as an integral aspect of his/her care throughout the course of the disease," and continues: "Not all cancer pain can be entirely eliminated, but available approaches, when appropriately and attentively applied, effectively relieve pain in most cases. The importance of effective pain management extends beyond [reducing or eliminating pain] to encompass the patient's quality of life and ability to function in the family and society."

The Washington State Pain Initiative Report of 1993 concludes that "although substantial numbers of cancer patients experience persistent pain . . . there appears to be little or no reason why that pain could not be effectively relieved by readily available and long-standing pain treatments. The World Health Organization (WHO) field trials and clinical experience have shown that 80% to 90% of cancer pain can be controlled/eliminated with minimal side effects by recommended WHO approaches."

Dr. R. K. Portnoy, an authority on the management of pain, observed in "Pain Control in the Patient with Cancer," a 1987 American Cancer Society pamphlet: "Expertise in pharmacologic [drugs] approaches alone could probably provide relief for at least 70% of cancer patients with pain, while a combination of several methods . . . can probably help most of the other 30%."

WHY IT IS SO IMPORTANT TO CONTROL PAIN

1. *Pain can make life a lot less pleasant.*
This needs no explanation.

2. *Pain depresses the immune system.*
John C. Liebeskind, Ph.D., of the UCLA Department of Psychology, in his 1991 article "Pain Can Kill" states: "Pain and stress can

inhibit immune function and enhance tumor growth . . . In humans severe, acute pain associated with surgery or trauma can also cause profound pathophysiological changes. Whether it is the pain itself or the stress reaction caused by the pain is still to be determined. However, it is clear that pain of sufficient magnitude can, directly or indirectly, suppress immune mechanisms normally serving to defend the body against tumors and can thereby cause a marked increase in tumor growth." In a later article in 1993, entitled "Morphine Attenuates Surgery-induced Enhancement of Metastatic Colonization in Rats," Dr. Liebeskind reports that experiments he conducted with rats suggest that "postoperative pain is a critical factor in promoting metastatic spread. If a similar relationship between pain and metastasis occurs in humans, then pain control must be considered a vital component of postoperative care."

3. *Pain can further weaken the patient.*
"Because pain diminishes activity, appetite and sleep, it can further weaken already debilitated patients." That statement appears in "Management of Cancer Pain," cited above.

4. *Pain removes the feeling of control in the patient.*
"Personal control is undermined when cancer is diagnosed and is further reduced by ongoing pain. . . . When pain reduces patients' options to exercise control, it diminishes psychological well-being and makes them feel helpless and vulnerable." ("Management of Cancer Pain")

ACTIONS YOU CAN TAKE TO CONTROL PAIN

STEP ONE:
Tell your physician about the pain and the degree of intensity. Sometimes it is easier to describe the intensity of the pain by placing a vertical line on the following horizontal line and showing that to your physician:

No pain	Little pain	Medium pain	Large pain	Worst Possible pain

STEP TWO:
If the pain does not abate, tell your doctor immediately.
Your physician wants to know so that he or she can do something
about it right away. Physicians are aware of just how debilitating
pain can be.

STEP THREE:
**While using the medication and ministrations for pain
as prescribed by your physician, also use the psychological
means available.**

PSYCHOLOGICAL TREATMENT
OF CANCER PAIN

As I said before, pain can be treated by medical, physical, or
psychological methods. Medical methods include drugs, operations, and treatments of like nature. Physical treatments include
the application of heat and cold, massage, pressure, or vibration.
The following is a short review of some of the mental methods you
can use. Each of the following psychological methods of pain
control and several others are well described in Dr. Jane Cowles's
book *Pain Relief, How to Say No to Acute, Chronic, and Cancer Pain,*
published in 1994 by Master Media.

The first is some form of relaxation such as Directed Visualization, discussed at some length in Chapter 9. You can also distract
yourself from the pain by laughter. In Chapter 10 I have discussed
that method in some detail. Purposely forcing yourself to think of
pleasant memories or anticipated events, either real or imagined,
and concentrating on counting the number of tiles on the walls or
the cars passing by are other methods of distraction.

One of my friends, who suffered severe pain from a sports

accident and the resulting operation, was involved with automobiles. The method he used to distract himself was to position himself where he could watch many cars go by and try to remember how many of each make he saw in a twenty-minute span. He said that he became quite good at it and that it distracted him enough that the pain did not seem to hurt as much.

Biofeedback, which is best provided by a person skilled in that form of assistance, is another possibility. What you are trying to do is distract your mind from paying attention to the pain. You can probably find such a person in your phone book.

ADDICTION FROM THE USE OF PAIN CONTROL DRUGS OCCURS ONLY RARELY

The scientists who study cancer pain are unanimous in their belief that fear of addiction is the main reason many cancer patients are reluctant to insist upon control of their pain. As is indicated by the statements set out below, such fear is unfounded. To understand more fully those statements, it's necessary that you understand the key words—"tolerance" to drugs, "dependence" on drugs, and "addiction." The U.S. Department of Health and Human Services ("Management of Cancer Pain," 1994) sets forth the following definitions:

- Addiction: the need to use drugs for *other than pain relief*
- Tolerance: a condition requiring a larger dose of a drug to maintain the same level of pain control
- Dependence: meaning that when the drug is discontinued the body has "flu-like" symptoms for a period of time

The Department of Health report further explains why the fear of addiction is unrealistic, in the following statements: "[Drug] tolerance and physical dependence are expected with long-term . . . treatment and should not be confused with . . .

addiction. [In almost all cases] there is no need for the use of any drug when the pain abates and therefore tolerance ceases to become an issue. In the same manner, there is usually no dependence on the drug after the drug is discontinued and there are no ill effects after the flu-like symptoms abate. The misunderstanding of these terms in relation to [drug] use leads to ineffective practices in prescribing, administering, and dispensing [drugs] for cancer pain and contributes to the problem of undertreatment. The presence of [drug] tolerance and physical dependence does not equate with 'addiction.' " Their final statement is: *"Physicians should reassure patients and families that most pain can be relieved safely and effectively. . . . Psychological dependence, addiction rarely if ever develops when narcotics are used for cancer pain. If the pain stops, the narcotics can be withdrawn safely and easily."*

In *Everyone's Guide to Cancer Therapy,* physicians E. H. Rosenbaum, Malin Dollinger, and Elliot Krames expose the myth about narcotics and cancer pain with the following statement: "Most cancer patients can take drugs for [pain], and only very rarely do they exhibit the drug abuse behaviors and psychological dependence that characterize addiction."

PATIENTS' FAILURE TO REPORT THEIR PAIN

Often cancer pain is not adequately treated because patients don't tell their doctors about the pain or the degree of it. The studies reveal the following reasons why patients are reluctant to communicate necessary information about pain.

1. Concern about distracting the physician from treatment of the underlying disease. Since many patients believe the pain is not causing any actual damage and the cancer is, they want their physician to concentrate on dealing with the progression of the disease and not be distracted by mere symptoms.

2. Belief that pain is a part of the disease and that it must be accepted as such.
3. Desire not to "bother" their physician with their pain.
4. Wish to appear "strong."

As you can see, none of those reasons makes very good sense. Tell your doctor when you are in pain. He or she wants to know and, because of all the foregoing, is intent on doing something about it.

CHAPTER 24

 c2—

You Don't Always Have to
Be Brave and Cheerful

The following story is a perfect illustration of how foolish the friends of cancer patients can be and what steps a very wise person took to protect herself from a well-meaning but foolish friend. This is the story of Marie, who had been fighting cancer for two years when I first met her at The Wellness Community. Marie had tried a support group before but had found it so depressing she dropped out after two meetings. She picked up the story by saying to a group we were both addressing, "When I first entered The Wellness Community, one of the first people I met and talked to was Harold Benjamin. We talked about the Patient Active concept and I decided to come to a Sharing Group and soon became an active participant in every part of the program."

To make clear the point of this anecdote, let me describe our meeting from my point of view. My first impression of Marie was of an attractive woman walking unsteadily with a cane, but whose unsure gait was overshadowed by her spirit. This spirit seemed to give a rosy glow to everything around her. Although she tells me now she was depressed, I never knew it.

Right from the beginning, whenever Marie was in the facility, she came to visit me—to tell me about her progress and what was going on in her life. But as time passed I saw her less and less frequently, although she was still coming to the Community as often as before. Wondering why, I asked the facilitator of Marie's group to ask her about it. Marie's explanation, which she authorized her facilitator to tell me, was: "Being with Harold became just too hard. He always expected me to be cheerful and energetic, when sometimes I just wanted to be tired old me. But I knew he wouldn't like me that way, so I just stayed away. I love Harold and I miss him, but being around him is just too difficult."

Marie was partly right and partly wrong. I would have liked to be with her even if she was tired and not so cheerful, but she didn't know that. I learned from that experience that many cancer patients, believing that their friends will turn away if they know how frightened, tired, or ill they really feel, always put on an act of being brave and cheerful, no matter how they feel. Their friends, in turn, also believe that the only "right" way to act with a cancer patient is to always be brave and cheerful. And it doesn't work.

My friend Marie was too smart to continue that charade, so she avoided me. She protected herself from what she saw as my demands. Somehow she knew that there are very few relationships that can survive the always-brave-and-cheerful syndrome, and that such forced gaiety places a tremendous strain on both parties. It can't be good for the patient's immune system.

But Marie was partly wrong. She didn't tell me what she saw as a problem. I would have changed. I did change when I knew what the problem was. I suggest that you tell your friends that sometimes you are not feeling well and want to be able to show that in their presence. After that, act brave and cheerful when you feel brave and cheerful or when you think acting that way is in your best interest, and when you don't—don't. I'm sure they will understand. This is no time to have the demands of others dictate how you will act. Do what you think is best for you. And know that you have a choice.

Just to finish the story—when I learned what was bothering Marie I talked to her about it and we became friends again. Marie and her family moved away about a year ago, and I still hear from her every once in a while.

So here are the "rules":

- Be brave and cheerful when you feel like it and civilized conduct demands it.
- Don't be brave and cheerful when you don't feel like it.
- Tell the people to whom you are not being brave and cheerful that you don't feel like being brave and cheerful, when you don't.
- Tell your friends not to demand that you be brave and cheerful all the time.
- Tell your friends that they don't have to be brave and cheerful all the time when they're around you.

The basic message is: Communicate, communicate, communicate.

CHAPTER 25

~?~

Use Upbeat Words About the Illness

You will notice in this chapter what appears to be a contradiction. In the previous chapter, I suggested that it may not be in your best interest to act brave and cheerful all the time, unless you are, and here I am advising that you use upbeat words about the illness even though you may not be feeling very well. That's not as confusing as it might seem, as you will understand as you read on.

I start this chapter with the understanding that what you are going through is truly unpleasant and deserving of graphic description. It's difficult not to complain when you have something to complain about. In times of discomfort we all want to describe the problem in terms that evoke a sympathetic response, and we deserve all the commiseration and understanding we can get. Being anxious about the future is an emotion that cries out for a sounding board: there is a part of us that knows that if someone understands and shares our apprehension, our anxiety will be reduced. And there is no question that there is a right time for complete candor and complaining to the right person. But, with cancer as part of the equation, should that be your primary method of communication with everyone, all the time?

Probably, before cancer, you chose your words based solely on the effect you wanted them to have on your listener without any thought that those words might also have an effect on you. But they do. So you might be wise to choose them carefully. Therefore, once again, you have a choice. You can describe the illness and its treatment and how they make you feel, using words and phrases that ensure that your listener understands every appalling nuance. Or you can choose to recount the experience in upbeat, more concise, down-to-earth terms, using less dramatic phrases and omitting some of the unpleasant details.

When making this decision you might ask yourself: "What effect do I want to evoke? Do I want my listeners to worry about me, feel sorry for me, or empathize with me? Do I want them to know how brave I am?" Nothing wrong with any of those motives. They are completely understandable. The more important question is: "What effect will the words, phrases, and tone of voice I use have on me?" The following will help you answer that question.

WHY THE WORDS YOU USE ABOUT THE ILLNESS ARE IMPORTANT

Words fix images and ideas in our minds, and if you use a word or a phrase, affect a certain demeanor, or use a certain tone of voice often enough, the point of view you are demonstrating may become a self-fulfilling prophecy. If you speak about the illness in funereal tones—if you call yourself a cancer victim or describe your bout with cancer as an ordeal or tell people you are suffering from a terminal or catastrophic illness—the certainty of an unpleasant future may implant itself not only in their minds but in yours. On the other hand, if you use more optimistic words, your body may hear a more hopeful prediction and react in a manner to assure a more desirable result.

If you give credence to the possibility that upbeat words are healthier than "downer words," the next question is, what upbeat and downer words are we talking about?

WHAT ARE DOWNER WORDS?

Before we get to the downer words, let's spend some time on the word "cancer." Here you will notice a switch. The advice of this chapter is to avoid using downer words, and although "cancer" is such a word, the advice is don't be afraid to use it. Many cancer patients are. We see that time after time at Wellness Community orientation meetings. At these meetings cancer patients new to The Wellness Community meet with others who have been participants in the program for some period of time and have recovered or are doing well with the illness. The people new to The Wellness Community say things like, "I have the big C," or they use some other euphemism as if saying "cancer" will bring to their consciousness just how serious their illness is.

But the veterans in the group use the word frequently and in context. They do this because they know that when "cancer" is used as part of ordinary conversation, while it never becomes just another word, it loses much of its frightening quality. Purposely avoiding the word imbues it with an ominous, almost superstitious quality.

Now we come to the downer words. The word "cancer" becomes frightening again when adjectives like "terminal," "catastrophic," or "deadly" are used to modify it, as in "terminal cancer." There's no reason to combine those words, and besides, in most cases it isn't accurate.

Additionally, people with cancer sometimes call themselves "cancer victims." Why? What purpose is served? Victims are helpless in the face of a specific adversity such as a tornado or a flood. So if you use the words "cancer victim," you are telling yourself, with every use of the phrase, that you are helpless—which, of course, is not true at all.

You'll find that the phrase "your illness" is never used in this book. After all, who would want to own cancer? Who would want to call the illness "my cancer"? You might ask yourself if you believe it's best to describe cancer as "invading" or "attacking"—what do those words indicate? Why use them?

UPBEAT WORDS

Upbeat words are difficult to describe because upbeatness about cancer is best indicated by your demeanor and by *not* using the downer words, phrases, or tone of voice. But there is an unusual set of circumstances here which must be considered. You may not believe it, but there is a group of people with cancer who, I believe unconsciously, are happiest when their friends and relations feel sorry for them. For them, using upbeat words or acting optimistic is counterproductive. That doesn't get them what they want. They know how to talk about hope, optimism, living life now, enjoying friends and fighting for recovery. They just don't want to do that. I mention this because it is possible that, without meaning to, you have fallen into that trap. For that reason, you might want to consider what reaction you want from the people you interact with and what words you are using to get that reaction.

Here is another situation where your friends can be helpful. Ask them the pertinent questions. See how they react. But, even if you don't want to do that, you can watch and see how you are acting. You can look inside and see what reaction you want. You can decide whether your demeanor is healthy for you.

I believe that the use of optimistic words will make you happier and perhaps have an effect on the course of the illness. However, you must decide whether you are happier having people feel sorry for you and deal with you as a cancer patient or having them react to you as the person you always were, except now you have cancer. The choice is yours.

WHAT ABOUT FRIENDS AND FAMILY WHO USE DOWNER WORDS?

Quite probably, your friends and family believe the same myths about cancer that you did. They don't know that there are millions of people to whom cancer is a memory and that there is plenty of room in life for love, laughter, and joy while fighting for recovery. They don't know that when they are downhearted they are depressing you. They think that the only way of relating to a person with cancer is to act dejected, discouraged, and dispirited. Their vocabulary is filled with words about the illness that we know are harmful. Well, don't let them do that to you. Tell them that they are depressing you. They will understand—so tell them. But remember, they don't have to be brave and cheerful all the time either. Life is complicated, isn't it?

The following is a story about Sharon, who came into one of our orientation meetings with a long face and drooping shoulders. She had been operated on five weeks before for colon cancer. Even though she had been told her prognosis was good, the words she used and her entire demeanor while describing her condition to us were those of a person who had no chance for survival. When the Orientation Group leaders brought that to her attention, Sharon seemed to resent their observations.

However, after she had heard several stories from others with cancer, her demeanor changed. We all watched it happen. As we were getting ready to leave, Sharon said, "I can't believe what I was doing. My doctor told me I would probably recover and yet I insisted on describing the illness I had as if it were terminal. I'm sure there was a part of me that felt I was terminal or I wouldn't have acted like that. I thank you for making me realize that. I don't feel terminal now. What a relief!"

Sharon's experience is enlightening. She unconsciously perpetuated an unrealistic perception by using words of doom and gloom. By paying attention to the words she used she became aware of this unconscious belief, so that she could take some action in regard to it. That's the point! That's what you might consider.

Remember what I said early in this book—that whatever you do is right for you? That is proven by the answers I received from Richard, who had lymphoma, and Lillian, who had breast cancer, when I spoke to them about the words they used to describe the illness. Here's what Richard said: "I never tell anyone how I feel— not my wife or my children, not even my group. I feel better when

I don't talk about how I feel. I don't hold back for the benefit of the listeners. I do it for me. Also, I told some of my friends not to ask me how I feel—and that works too. I just don't want to talk about it."

Then there's Lillian, who fought breast cancer for several years. Here's what she said: "When I was first diagnosed, my group told me that I was constantly describing my 'suffering' in the most awful terms and they suggested that I consider trying something else. Well, I started to tell only my husband how I really felt and even with him I was careful about the words I used. I didn't want to make it worse than it really was. With everyone else, I talked about how I felt as if it wasn't as bad as it really was. That wasn't so easy in the beginning because I was sick most of the time and, for whatever reason, I wanted to tell everyone how lousy I felt—but I didn't. I must also admit that when I felt reasonably well, I wasn't anxious to tell anyone about that phase of my illness—but I did. Strangely enough, it made me feel better. Also, my friends didn't pity me and that helped. Now it's a good deal easier because I have been without symptoms or treatment for several months and I feel well. I would recommend that everyone think about how they talk about their illness. The change made a world of difference for me."

ANOTHER REASON TO USE UPBEAT WORDS

There is a second benefit of using more hopeful words. That benefit is based on the fact that your subconscious has a great deal of difficulty remembering the sensations and emotions you feel, but has no difficulty at all remembering forever every word of your description of those sensations. The memory of an emotion is amorphous and soon disappears. The description of the emotion remains for a much longer time. For instance, if after chemo-therapy you describe the treatment and your reaction to it, making sure that your listener knows just how awful you feel, your mem-ory of the nausea will be, for a very long time, that sickening feeling you described. Conversely, if you talk as if the chemo and the nausea were not all that bad, perhaps, at least in part, what you will remember is the "not so bad" description. So, because you know that how you describe the experience will determine to some extent how you remember it, you might want to give some thought to that description.

It is the consensus of my colleagues and me, based on our interactions with hundreds of cancer patients who have reacted adversely to chemotherapy, that those who describe the experience as tolerable rather than intolerable seem to be less anxious about future treatments than those who are more graphic in their descriptions. These observations are clearly anecdotal and not the basis of a formal examination. Additionally, there *is* the possibility that those who used the bland words actually had a less traumatic experience. However, what have you got to lose by using upbeat words except the sympathy of your listener?

A THIRD REASON TO USE UPBEAT WORDS

Finally, the third reason for downplaying unpleasant feelings and sensations is the effect the constant reiteration of those feelings and sensations have on your companions. When you were well, did you want to listen to someone who frightened you or depressed you all the time? I believe that makes the point!

CHAPTER 26

Don't Be Too Nice

There is the notion, believed by many professionals, that being too nice can suppress the immune system and therefore negatively affect the course of the illness when cancer is already present. This information is all quite recent. The first scientific observation that withholding anger and hostility might have an adverse effect on physical well-being was made in the 1950s. The world is moving at a very fast pace.

WHAT DOES BEING "TOO NICE" MEAN?

In 1993, Lydia Temoshok, Ph.D., wrote *The Type C Connection*, in which she described Type C personalities as those who ". . . coped by keeping their feelings under wraps. They never expressed anger and rarely did they express fear and sadness. They maintained a facade of pleasantness even under the most painful and aggravating circumstances. They strived excessively to please [others]." In other words—they are too nice. The behavior of these too nice people is that they don't express anger or hostility; their main purpose seems to be making sure that others like them, even at the cost of extreme self-sacrifice; they are ultrapatient, cooperative, and seek to avoid confrontation under all circumstances.

Of course, I know many cancer patients who aren't nice at all. So it must be understood that not everybody who is too nice develops cancer and not everyone who develops cancer is too nice.

CAN BEING TOO NICE AFFECT
THE COURSE OF THE ILLNESS?

The answer is yes—it might. Dr. Temoshok came to the conclusions that "our physical health is compromised when we chronically repress our needs and feelings to accommodate others . . . [and that] this coping style weakens our immune defenses and leaves us more vulnerable to cancer progression." In the late 1970s, C. B. Bahnson, Ph.D., found that an inordinate number of cancer patients have a "personality marked by self-containment, inhibition, rigidity, repression, and regression." At about the same time, Lawrence LeShan, Ph.D., observed that many cancer patients are described by friends as being "too good to be true, gentle, fine, thoughtful, and uncomplaining." He wrote, "Cancer patients appear to be compliant, submissive, passive, selfless, and anxious to please in order to avoid being disliked." My own observation is that within The Wellness Community I have met a disproportionate number of our participants who are so nice as to be hard to believe.

The important questions for you are: "Am I too nice? Am I a Type C personality?" If you are, the next question is: "Can this personality trait be modified?" Dr. Temoshok believes that it can, and I agree with her. She says that "any therapy or process that helps patients change Type C behavior will strengthen their recovery process." I would say it another way. I believe that excessively repressing or suppressing one's true feelings as a dominant coping mechanism can have a negative effect on the immune system, and that becoming aware of that damaging coping mechanism and taking some action to modify it may have a positive effect on the immune system, and therefore may alter the course of the illness toward health.

The purpose of this chapter is to suggest methods by which you can become aware of whether you use that damaging coping mechanism, and if you do, some actions you can use to change.

But first you must determine whether or not you are "too

nice." If, after honest introspection, you determine that you are always agreeable, always helpful, always friendly and courteous, and are not repressing or covering up some other emotion such as anger, frustration, or hostility—go for it! You are not too nice, you are just nice. And very unusual.

If, on the other hand, you find that by always being nice you are suppressing negative feelings, you probably should do something about it. And whatever you do should probably be done in baby steps. Parenthetically, "repression" means that the individual is unaware of the unpleasant feelings. "Suppression" means that the individual knows of the unpleasant feelings but hides them.

SPECIFIC ACTIONS YOU CAN TAKE

STEP ONE:

To determine if you are being too nice, ask yourself questions such as these: "Was I too nice today? Was I pleasant and helpful to John when he hasn't ever been nice to me and what I really wanted to do was to tell him to get lost? Did I listen to Lois give me advice about my illness when I know she doesn't know what she's talking about and all I wanted her to do was leave me alone?" These questions will force you to shift to the left hemisphere of your brain to consider whether your actions coincided with your desires and objectively determine whether you were being too nice or only nice.

We all do nice things for other people even though we would rather be doing something else. Nothing unusual or harmful about that. The Type C personality carries it to the extreme.

STEP TWO:

If you believe you are acting too nice too often, watch for the next situation where you are in conflict—where you are acting nice when you want to act in another way—and take a chance. Take a chance that people will still love you even though you're not a saint. Do it because you believe it's good for you. What you are really doing is *acting as if* (see Chapter 8).

STEP THREE:

Don't go too far. It's probably just as bad to be a curmudgeon as to be too nice. This is not an easy task. I believe it is often more difficult for the nice guy to become normal than for the tough guy to become nice. There is a middle ground. Seek it as part of your fight for recovery.

CHAPTER 27

∾

Expect the Best

The suggestion is broader than the title. It includes *not only* using optimistic words about cancer (see Chapter 25), maintaining hope (see Chapter 11), making plans for the future (see Chapter 28) *but also* attempting to think of the future in terms of recovery. With this advice, I must be careful that you do not understand me to be encouraging false hope or ignoring the facts. That's certainly not my intention. What I am suggesting is that you act as if you expect to be in the percentage of those people who have recovered from the same cancer you have. There is always a percentage who recover. Once again, I have presented you with a choice. You can choose to *think of yourself as part of the group who will recover or as part of the group of those who won't.* I hope you chose the former. I hope I would choose the former. *I know you can't change a life-long method of reacting to life events by just deciding to do it. It's a difficult task and takes work and concentration. But it's worth a try and just trying will have a positive effect.*

There are at least four excellent reasons for envisioning the future as optimistically as you can: The first is that anticipating the future with optimism is likely to bring an immediate warm glow—a pleasant emotion, which, as we well know, enhances the immune system. The second is that if you expect the best, you may galvanize the placebo effect, which was described in Chapter 21. The third is that those who expect a favorable result are happier than those with a gloomy expectation—and I'm sure you will agree, happy is better than sad. The fourth has to do with the thesis known as self-fulfilling prophecy, which augurs well for the patient who expects to recover.

That thesis suggests that if we believe in the inevitability of a certain result, we will act either consciously or unconsciously to ensure the expected result. One example is the cancer patient mentioned in Chapter 21 who took a worthless drug called Krebiozen, and because he expected it to cure him, it did. Another example is of the witch doctor who prophesies that a particular tribal member will die at a given time, and turns out to be right. It is quite possible that the reason for the death as prophesied is that the unfortunate victim so believed in the inevitability of the prophecy that he unconsciously instructed his body to die at the appointed hour. In essence, this is the placebo effect in reverse and a perfect example of the self-fulfilling prophecy.

Various researchers have applied this thesis to cancer patients, theorizing that people who expect to recover are more likely to do so than individuals who believe there is no hope for recovery. Robert K. Menon, Ph.D., an authority on the subject, has written that "the self-fulfilling prophecy is, in the beginning, a *false* definition of a situation, evoking a new behavior which makes the originally false definition come true." Dr. Menon observed: "If a cancer patient expects the illness to be one from which he can recover, which may be against all of the odds (a false premise), perhaps he unconsciously directs his body to fight even harder and this new behavior results in the outcome he prophesied— recovery."

Thus, you see that you may benefit by having as many positive expectations and as few negative expectations as possible. Of course, you cannot change an expectation by the stroke of an intention; but many cancer patients have changed from believing that their illness is fatal to believing and hoping that recovery is a definite possibility. They have achieved this with the help of their friends and other cancer patients, and by using the "act as if" technique described in Chapter 8.

Ryan, forty-five, who has been recovered from colon cancer

for over twelve years, is an example of a cancer patient who went from pessimism to optimism and believes that change had an effect on the course of the illness. He says: "When I heard I had colon cancer, my doctors told me to get my affairs in order, since my time was quite limited. And I believed them. With all my heart and soul, I believed them. I went through the operation and the treatment but I was sure it was a waste of time. For several weeks my group had been telling me that my pessimism was getting in my way, but I didn't listen to them. I knew I was going to die. But one morning I woke up and decided that I wasn't going to give up without a fight. Even though I believed I was going to die, because they told me so, I decided that recovery was a possibility and that I was going to do everything I could to make that happen. And, although I had always been a very private person, I went right downstairs and announced this to my wife and children. I also told all my friends that I knew that the treatments I was receiving were going to cure me. I kept saying this over and over again, even when I felt as sick as a dog. After a while, every time I talked about my recovery—and I would talk about it a lot—I would feel a thrill of hope run through me. I also started to talk about my plans for the future, even though there was a part of me that 'knew' I was kidding myself. And the more I talked about the future the more possible it seemed that there would be a future for me. I don't know if that had anything to do with my recovery, but it sure made me feel better."

As I report on Ryan's case I am concerned that you will believe that if you can be as good and as diligent as Ryan, you are sure to recover—that all you have to do is learn to do it right, and if you are trying these methods and they don't work, it's your fault. That's just not true. You are doing it, whatever "it" is, as well as it can be done.

But there is the possibility that what you do, feel, and think will have an effect on the course of the illness, and it doesn't make sense to hide or ignore those who have recovered just because we are concerned about the issue of false hope. Discussing the cases of recovery creates no problem just so long as we understand that the methods suggested do not always work, that if they don't seem to be working it's not your fault, that whatever you are doing is perfect, and that sometimes biology is stronger than psychology. That's the fine line we must walk.

Why don't you stop reading now and think about the ways you would act, the plans you would make, and the things you would say if you expected to recover. Then go out and say them and do them. That's "acting as if," and it may just trigger your immune system into working as hard as it can for your recovery. This does not preclude discussing your fears and anxieties—but why dwell on your doubts? What good will that do?

Don't be discouraged if results take a while. However, if you've given this approach a full try and it doesn't work, don't blame yourself. It doesn't work for everybody. Try something else.

Expectations can also be important in dealing with your treatment. If you expect chemotherapy to cause nausea and vomiting, it probably will. Many cancer patients become ill on the way to the doctor's office at the mere thought of the treatment. It's interesting to note that although cancer is the enemy and chemotherapy is a friend, they are painted with the same hateful brush. But just as the body reacts negatively to a negative thought, perhaps it will react positively to the thought that you will have no nausea from the treatment. Try to view the treatment as an aid to recovery, not as an enemy. You might also want to meditate, using visualization techniques, before, during, and after chemotherapy or radiation.

Take the case of Geoff, who decided to act as if the radiation treatments he was receiving for brain cancer were "friends with magical properties," in the hope that doing so would help the treatment achieve its maximum effectiveness and minimize its side effects. This change in his attitude did not evolve unconsciously; it was a decision carefully arrived at, after he had been advised that such a step might be helpful. He considered the advice, saw he had nothing to lose, and decided to accept it.

Geoff then started to think and speak of his treatments not as horrendous, dreadful times of torture with awful sickness and nausea as the inevitable result; instead, he spoke as if they were a method of fighting for recovery that had only irritating, not sickening, side effects. And gradually, his perception of the treatment changed. The unpleasant effects diminished. This won't happen to everyone, but it's worth a try.

Cassandra provides another example of expectations coming to fruition. She fought breast cancer for several years and has been symptom-free for many years. She always considered chemotherapy her friend and ally, picturing it as a vat of liquid that would disintegrate unhealthy cells to make room for healthy ones. And it never made her sick. Maybe it wouldn't have under any circumstances, but Cassandra likes to think that her attitude had something to do with the way she reacted to her treatment, and perhaps her prophecy of recovery was self-fulfilling. And perhaps—just perhaps—you can experience the same results.

CHAPTER 28

～

Make Plans for the Future

If you are not making plans for the future, it may be because you don't see any future in your future. You may have *unconsciously* given up, and that can have serious consequences. Here, I am not discussing the possibility that you have *consciously* given up or no longer want to fight, which is a matter worthy of its own book. I am discussing the possibility that you have *unconsciously* given up because you *unconsciously* believe that there is no chance of recovery. If you believe that, you may, without meaning to, be instructing your body not to work so hard—that no matter what it does, it won't make any difference. That, of course, is exactly the opposite of what you want your mind to tell your body.

Stop now and think about it. Do you believe there is a future for you, or are you resigned to the fact that there is no way that you can recover? I can't think of a more important question you can ask yourself. If the answer is that you expect to recover or that there is a chance of your recovery, from my point of view that's the way it should be. If, however, there is significant doubt in your mind, there are some steps you might take.

I could suggest that you merely change your mind-set, but that's unrealistic. I don't know the mechanism for that type of radical change. But I do know a trick. The trick is—make plans for the future. There are at least three reasons for consciously making plans for a trip two years from now or for how you will spend the next several New Year's Days or be around to see all of your children have children. First, making plans is fun. Second, you may be countermanding a giving-up instruction you have unconsciously given to your body. Think about that. It's an interesting and convoluted concept. Assume that Mrs. Jones has unconsciously given up. Based on all the facts she knows, all the myths she believes, and her total life experience, she is convinced that there is no hope. We agree that it's difficult, if not impossible, for her to just turn that around and tell herself that there is at least a chance of recovery. However, if she starts to plan for the future, she bypasses the myths and beliefs and takes action—gives orders to her psyche—as if those myths and beliefs were no longer controlling. Her psyche may deal with the concept of the future plans without reference to the unpleasant myths and beliefs.

The third reason to make plans for the future is that you may be instructing your body to do everything it can to be around when that day comes, and there's precedent that your body may comply with those instructions.

Haven't we all watched and heard about people with a limited prognosis who outlived that prognosis so that they could attend a wedding, a graduation, or see their grandchild? Why did that happen? How did those people extend their lives by sheer force of will? Cynics hold that they would have lived that long no matter what they did. Perhaps so. However, several professionals with whom I have spoken believe that there is the real possibility that those people instructed their bodies to survive until that date and their bodies complied. Perhaps you can give your body the same instructions.

Take heart. The results of making plans for the future are probably more accessible to you than they were to the people we all heard about. The reason we find those stories so remarkable is that the people in question were at death's door when they instructed their bodies to hold on. They held off the Grim Reaper even though they had an extremely weak constitution to work with. You are probably not in so desperate a condition. If they could stimulate their immune systems and the rest of their bodies to such herculean efforts in their desperate condition, isn't it even more likely that you can do the same in your less serious condition?

There are those who argue that making plans for the future for the purposes discussed above is dangerous in that, since the people in question died soon after the event occurred, maybe they had programmed their bodies to die rather than to live. So, my advice is to make many and continuing plans for the future—not just one. That's exactly what you did when you were well. Don't stop now.

CHAPTER 29

⌒୨—

Don't Keep Secrets

I suggest that you keep as few secrets as possible because, as you will see, each secret you keep requires the expenditure of energy you can use fighting to get well. Such secret-keeping energy is expended by the necessity of being ever alert and watchful lest you let that secret slip out by something you say or do. Stop now and think about a secret you are keeping and examine how much effort you put into making sure no one knows it. I believe that if you are truthful with yourself, you are in for a big surprise.

I certainly don't suggest that you tell every secret about yourself—obviously, there are some facts it makes good sense to keep private. But I do suggest that you consciously decide which secrets are worth using the energy for, and which you should let go. To help make that determination, we should first look at what secrets are about and why we keep them.

We keep secrets about what we believe we have done wrong or something we believe to be shameful—about our physical or mental makeup, our heritage, what we hope for the future, what our desires are, etc., etc. And we keep those secrets because we "know" that if someone knew that secret, we would get in trouble or "they" wouldn't like us, wouldn't respect us, wouldn't let us in their club, wouldn't do what we want them to. Both lists could go on forever.

My experience is that we keep many of our secrets for foolish reasons—reasons which, if brought to conscious consideration, don't make any sense at all. An illustration of that is Charles, a Wellness Community participant who had been a friend of mine for many years. He had testicular cancer and was determined to do everything he could to make sure that his life would go on much as it had been before the diagnosis.

I knew, because he had told me and many of our mutual friends, that he was born in a large eastern city and had lived there until he was about fifteen in modest financial circumstances. One afternoon, he called and asked if I would meet him for lunch—he had something that his group suggested he tell me because we were old friends. I could not imagine what it was. I had all kinds of fantasies about dramatic events in his life or his relationships with his wife and children. What he told me blew me away. He revealed with difficulty that, as a boy, he had not lived in modest comfort but had lived above a store in a very poor neighborhood and his family was in the most dire financial circumstances. Who cared?

Upon hearing that, I was shocked—not because it made the slightest difference to me where Charles had lived as a boy but because I could see no reason for keeping the secret and, more important, because of the amount of stress he had placed on himself to keep that dumb secret: He had to be sure that the friends he made as an adult, like me, never met any of his old friends. When we reminisced about our childhoods, he had to either lie or carefully skirt the truth. He was under constant strain about a secret that didn't make any difference at all. Now that he had let the cat out of the bag, he didn't have to worry about that any longer. What a relief!

Here's the important part. I believe we all have secrets much like Charles's—that nobody cares about. Why don't you check and see if you agree with me. The way to do that is to make a list of the secrets you keep. You might start by asking yourself questions like the following: "What have I done that I am keeping secret? What am I ashamed of that I am keeping secret?" Those are just for starters.

It may take a lot of thought to make your list, because most of us keep secrets we don't know we are keeping—they are buried very deep. But stick to it. You have nothing to lose, and you may gain a lot. By the way, when I decided to make a list of my secrets, I had no difficulty at all. My "secrets" spewed out in a torrent. I told mine to a group of friends. Obviously, I had unconsciously been waiting for the opportunity.

The immediate benefits of the list are twofold—first, you will know that you have secrets and what they are, and second, by listing them you will define and separate the secrets one from another, so that you can look at each one and decide whether you ought to keep it secret. That way, you won't have to consider them all at once, which is impossible to do.

One Patient Active, a university professor with lung cancer, had the following experience: "When I first joined my group, everything in my life was a secret. I have always been a very private person. But soon I saw that not much was happening for me in the group, while some of the others who told a lot more about themselves seemed to be having a lot more fun. So I took a chance. I told them that I had failed several courses in high school. That had always been something I hid. I don't think I even knew I was hiding it. I guess I believed that if they knew about my failure, they wouldn't think I was as smart as I wanted them to. When I revealed that secret, and told them that even my wife didn't know about it, even I saw how foolish it was. With that experience under my belt, I became bolder and bolder, and it became easier and easier to tell more about myself. The funny thing is that the more they knew about me the more they seemed to like me, and the better I felt about myself. People don't like or dislike you because of what you tell them. They make that decision based on how you treat them."

To determine whether your reasons for keeping secrets are rational, consider each one on your list and ask yourself why you can't discuss it with your friends. Will they like or respect you less? Be realistic. If the tables were turned and they revealed such a secret to you, how would you react? If your reason for keeping the secret turns out to be reasonable, then keep it. But if not, don't. It takes too much energy.

CHAPTER 30

❧

Continue to Enjoy Sex
and Intimacy

Problems of sexuality and intimacy are not unusual when cancer is the diagnosis. Experience suggests that if such problems are a part of your life they are probably due to your cancer-related inability to participate in sex or intimacy as you did before, a decrease in your desire to be sexual or intimate, or both. *Take heart—ability and libido almost always reappear as the stress or treatment decreases.* It's important that you integrate that fact into your belief system because if you do, much of the anxiety about the future of your sex life will be eliminated. But even with your new perception of the future, there still remains the lack of warmth and physical affection during your fight for recovery. The remedies you might try for that state of affairs are described and examined in this chapter.

Some of the specific physical conditions that may inhibit intimacy and decrease sexual desire are listed here so that you will know you are not unusual if you experience one or more of them. They include reduced response to touch, reduced stamina, fatigue, and pain. Additionally, intercourse may be out of the question either because physical changes make it impossible, or because it's medically inadvisable. Also, sex sometimes disappears from the patient's life because of psychological reactions to cancer. They include the patient's belief that he or she is no longer desirable, the pervasive fear of the future, or the partner's belief that the patient is unwilling or unable to participate in sex or intimacy.

I believe, along with many of my colleagues, that the most

important tool for solving these problems, both mental and physical, is communication, which all too often is missing between the cancer patient and his or her partner. The following scenario is not unusual: The cancer patient doesn't want to broach the subject of sex or intimacy because he's afraid she won't want to fondle or sleep with someone who has cancer or whose body has changed so radically. At the same time, the well partner is reluctant to make any advances toward intimacy out of concern that the cancer patient's libido is diminished, since most of his energy is spent fighting the illness. Who will speak first? What will happen if neither speaks? Answer: If neither speaks, nothing will happen. That's the point! If neither speaks, nothing will happen.

For most people, sex is a difficult subject to deal with under the best of circumstances; with cancer, feelings of sexual inadequacy or insecurity can become greatly magnified. However, it is commonly understood by those who specialize in this field that most intimacy problems can be satisfactorily dealt with—but they must not be ignored. If the problem is to be resolved you must communicate. If your partner seems reluctant to participate in intimacy—ask the questions important to you, questions like, "Why have you been avoiding intimacy since the diagnosis?" and, "Should we try to be as intimate as we were before the diagnosis?" *The imagined answers to unasked questions keep many of us on edge nearly all the time; for cancer patients, such uncertainty is even more serious.* Make your desires known: "I would like to be as intimate as we were before; however, we must be careful because [put in the reason and the area where care must be taken]." *Dare to communicate clearly about what you would like, physically as well as emotionally.* If you learn only this lesson from this chapter, it will be enough. Everything else will fall into place. This advice is not always easy to follow. *However, if you decide not to start the conversation because you fear the worst, then you'd better resign yourself to fantasy, because fantasy is all you're going to get.*

The experience of George can be helpful here. George was fifty-one and had been cancer-free for many years when I met him. He came to a meeting on sexuality at The Wellness Community so that others could benefit from his experience. Here's what George said.

I had colon cancer and a colostomy. I hated it. I'm still not too fond of it but I know it was and is a part of saving my life. I was about thirty-six and had been married for almost five years when all this happened. We had one child and a fair sex life. We had planned to have more children. While I was still in treatment, I never felt very well and often I felt downright sick, and besides that, I knew I might die, so I wasn't much interested in sex. It didn't seem that Harriet was either. She had problems of her own, many caused by my illness. That went on for about two years. When I knew I was going to live, my libido started to return but I was afraid to make the advance. After two years of abstinence, I wasn't sure of the response I would get. Besides that, the damned thing seemed to me to be always smelly. Who would want to sleep with a guy with that thing on? So I never made the approach and that went on for another two years. I was resigned to never having sex again and I wasn't happy.

One afternoon, I received a call from my dearest friend—an accountant. He asked to see me at his office on an urgent matter. I rushed to his office thinking there was a problem with the I.R.S., and when I walked in, there was Harriet. Harriet had told Arthur about our no-sex life and wanted to talk. Smart girl, Harriet. The talk lasted about two minutes because as soon as I knew she was interested and she knew I was interested, Arthur was no longer important. We left Arthur, went home, and decided that before we would take the next step we would call the surgeon who operated on me to see what could be done about the bag during sex. To come to the point, we now have a second child and a basic understanding of the fact that although talk is cheap, without it you can miss a great deal in life.

But keep in mind that sex doesn't necessarily mean sexual intercourse. It can mean touching, cuddling, stroking, brushing the hair, a kiss or a massage. It can be any sign of intimate affection given with love and the mutual need to be physically close. But although it's possible that the parties will discover these alternate methods of showing love by chance, the risk that the discovery won't be made is substantially reduced by open and loving communication.

If your partner has taken the lead and reestablished the sexual relationship, you don't have a problem. But if not, although it may frighten you silly you can be the one to indicate a desire for romantic involvement. With the right response, your sex life together can return to where it was before, or close to it. But if you don't take the initiative, your partner may also be unwilling to initiate the conversation, and intimacy may be indefinitely delayed or forgotten.

All of the foregoing is based on the assumption that both partners want to reestablish a sexual relationship. Suppose, however, that your significant other is actually put off by the change in your body or the onset of the illness. You should know this as soon as possible, and the only way you will really know is if you ask. Since there is the possibility that this might change with time, there is no alternative but to be patient and see how matters develop. But if your partner's feelings don't change I'm afraid that you have no alternative but to accommodate to the situation or terminate the relationship. Some sexual problems brought about by cancer are so complex as to require the help of a psychiatrist, psychologist, clinical social worker, or marriage and family therapist. Sometimes your physician can help.

One word of caution before I make specific suggestions. Cancer can bring about feelings of selfishness and self-involvement that foreclose all emotions except the desire for recovery. But suppose—because you believe your partner wants and needs sex and intimacy—even though you do not feel sexual, you are doing what you feel is necessary. If you know why you are doing it and don't resent it, that's okay. But if you do resent it, that feeling will fester and taint the relationship, perhaps forever. So, if the latter is your situation, you had better bring it out in the open as soon as possible, and whatever happens will be better than what will happen if the matter is left unexamined. You will be interested to know that most of the cancer patients with whom I discussed this matter believe that you, as a cancer patient, have no obligation to be involved in intimacy if you don't feel well enough.

I will now suggest some specific methods you can use to deal with the immediate lack of warmth and affection brought about by cancer. I do so with the understanding that both you and your partner are interested in some type of intimate activity. However, if that's not the case, and sex is no longer an issue to either of you, at least while the fight for recovery continues, then go on to another chapter.

THE PAIN PROBLEM

Even if you are in pain most of the time, sex is not necessarily out of the question if you don't want it to be. If there are periods in the day or in the cycle of treatments when you feel better, you can plan intimacy for those times and have something to fantasize about and look forward to.

A good time for shared intimacy may be after taking pain medication or after meditation and relaxation exercises. If you are still too uncomfortable for intercourse at these times, you may be able to participate in gentler types of sexual activity, like massage or stimulating the sexual organs with oils or lotions.

If a scar is tender, try placing a pillow near the site of the incision or beneath it. Experiment with different positions until you come up with ones that put the least amount of weight or pressure on you. "Spoons" is one such position, where the couple lie side by side like spoons cradled one in the other. The best method for

making accommodations and new discoveries is to visualize, fantasize, and discuss them with your partner. Then try them.

THE FATIGUE FACTOR

It is not uncommon for cancer patients to feel tired most of the
time. And fatigue inhibits sexuality. Our participants often deal
with this problem by involving themselves in some less energetic
activity, such as hugging, caressing, taking a shower together, or
rubbing each other with oils.

However, while such foreplay might be good for you, it may
not satisfy the partner who isn't too tired to be aroused. In those
circumstances, you might consider satisfying your partner in some
way that is not too physically demanding. You can plan this kind of
intimacy for times when you have just rested, meditated, or had a
full night's sleep.

THE BODY IMAGE ADJUSTMENT

Adjusting to a body change is sometimes the most difficult aspect
of the illness. It takes time, effort, and thought to accept and
integrate this new and unalterable part of your life. But if you don't
spend this time and effort, your new condition may relegate you to
feeling unlovable and untouchable, perhaps forever.

The key here is to acknowledge your feelings. Talk about those
feelings—don't ignore them. After an operation, many cancer
patients hide the scar from their partner. But if the relationship is
ever to be intimate and comfortable, such hiding cannot go on
forever. Since it is inevitable that your partner will see the scar
sooner or later, make sure that you pick the time and place for the
unveiling. Whether you do it with humor, solemnity, or something
in between is up to you. However, be aware that your attitude can
be the most significant factor in your partner's accommodation. If

you see the bodily change as a romance-ending catastrophe, your partner may have difficulty seeing it as anything else.

None of this is easy. No one can tell you what will work for you. But one universal truth seems to emerge—the best chance of a happy ending comes from telling each other the truth in a loving and caring way.

PHYSICAL INABILITY

When temporary or permanent bodily changes make it difficult or impossible to receive or give pleasure as you did before, other methods must be found. Some solutions are described in *Sexual Side Effects of Cancer,* written by Marion E. Morra of the Yale Comprehensive Cancer Center and published by the National Cancer Institute:

> Genital intercourse is only one way of expressing physical love. People find that using hands, thumbs, fingers, tongues, lips, mouth, and anal areas may provide exciting and pleasurable alternatives to penile-vaginal intercourse. Intra-thigh and intra-mammary (placing the penis between the thighs or between the breasts) may also be an option. All these options are "normal sex." . . . Masturbation is a form of sexual activity that can be a satisfactory alternative form of gratification when sexual intercourse is not possible or not desired . . . Some women have found that mechanical vibrators can be used, either by themselves or along with other sexual activities with their partners.

But nothing can take place without communication. Everything changes when partners tell each other what gives them the most pleasure. And partners can guide each other's hands to the areas of pleasure and indicate how hard or soft they want the pressure there to be. That's communication too.

SPECIAL NEEDS OF THE CANCER PATIENT
ENTERING INTO A NEW RELATIONSHIP

How to tell a potential sexual partner that you have cancer is the purpose of this section. How do you tell a potential partner that the illness or its treatment has left you with only one breast, with an ostomy bag, or unable to have an erection? When do you make these facts known?

The mere fact that you have cancer will be enough to make it impossible for some people to have a long-term relationship with you. They just aren't going to let themselves fall in love with someone who is facing cancer-related problems, and both of you should know that as soon as possible. While you should probably not open a conversation by saying, "Hello, my name is John [or Jane] Smith and I have cancer," you should make the fact known as soon as you see the relationship starting to move in the direction of permanency, because sooner or later, the information is going to come out.

This early communication is the only fair way to deal with the situation, and it will also protect you from being hurt more deeply than need be. If the other person is going to move away, let it be before you become more involved. All kinds of rationalizations can be made for withholding the information, but the consensus is—the sooner the better.

The question of how you convey the information has only one answer: Say it straight out. For instance, "John [Jane], I find that I'm looking forward to seeing you more and more, and it seems to me that you are becoming more interested in me. Because of that, I want you to know that I have [or have had] cancer." The conversation will go on from there.

As far as bodily changes are concerned, your potential partner is going to find out about them as soon as intimacy begins. *Don't let the discovery of this bodily change come as a shock at a time of arousal.* If he is reaching for a breast that isn't there, or she suddenly realizes you are wearing some type of ostomy bag, your partner may say or exclaim something for which you both will be sorry. Tell your partner about the bodily change under neutral, nonaroused circumstances, so that he or she will have time to ask questions and accept the information. If that information makes the relationship impossible, you'd better find out—the sooner the better.

YOUR PARTNER'S NEED FOR INTIMACY

This section of the book is the only one addressed to someone other than you. I include it so that you can share it with your sexual partner if you feel it will be helpful.

Recently, I asked several partners of Wellness Community participants to describe the emotions they were experiencing related to sex. The emotion that surfaced most often was guilt over their need for sex while their partner was so ill. The partners also confessed to guilt after having intercourse, convinced that their partner did it just to oblige them. After discussion, however, the group agreed on the following: (1) Guilt related to one's sexual needs after one's partner is diagnosed with cancer is unrealistic, unnecessary, and easily dispensed with if the parties talk to each other. (2) The cancer patient *should* make a *reasonable* effort to meet his or her partner's sexual needs. What is reasonable and how that should be done will be revealed by open discussions, with the specific knowledge that there are many methods available to satisfy the need for intimacy which take little or no effort on the part of the cancer patient. (3) All the needs of both parties can and will be met with communication.

CHAPTER 31

Know You Are Not to Blame
for the Onset of the Illness

To blame yourself for the onset of the illness is not only unrealistic but silly. That thought, the possibility that the patient may be responsible for the onset of the illness, is of very recent vintage. It serves no purpose to discuss the origin of this belief. But wherever it came from, it's wrong! It's wrong and it's dangerous. The only mind-set I can think of that is more debilitating than believing that you brought the cancer on yourself is to believe that you are not recovering as fast as you should because of something you are doing wrong. Both of these beliefs are sheer nonsense. In the next chapter I will discuss the "I am at fault for not recovering as fast as I should" nonsense. Here, we will discuss the "I brought the cancer on myself" nonsense.

It's true that your lifestyle and coping mechanisms may have had a debilitating effect on your immune system, but how were you to know that? When cancer patients come to The Wellness Community with that belief, they soon learn that in order to be at fault for the onset of the illness, they would have had to continue acting in a way that could cause cancer after they actually knew such actions could have that result. As soon as this subject comes up, they are asked: "Did you, prior to the diagnosis, have the slightest notion that the way you were living and reacting to life events might cause cancer?" Unless the issue is smoking or excessive sunbathing, the answer is invariably no. Only if they *knew* they were risking cancer by some action and did it anyway can they blame themselves. And even then they can't really be sure that if they had acted differently, the results would have been different.

Think back before the diagnosis. Can you remember even one occasion when you thought that the way you were acting might be weakening your immune system or was exposing you to cancer? If not, then blaming yourself for the disease is at best unrealistic and at worst dangerous—dangerous because the resulting feelings of inadequacy and guilt may exacerbate your stress.

If you blame yourself, you may trigger two other self-defeating reactions. You may unconsciously forgo taking actions in your fight for recovery, and you may inhibit the spontaneous self-healing responses your body would automatically take to return to its normal condition.

If you have cancer and blame yourself, this would be a good time to ask yourself the following questions. Consider each one carefully.

- Do you believe that you are to blame or responsible for the onset of the disease? (If your answer is yes, try to define exactly what you did or didn't do that caused or failed to prevent the disease.)
- Are you sure that different actions on your part would have altered the course of the disease?
- Did you fail to take some action that you, at that time, believed would prevent cancer from developing?
- Did you know that the way you were living and coping with the problems of life might be making you more vulnerable to the development of cancer?

I have never known anyone who even though he blamed himself for the disease could remember an occasion when he did or failed to do something while *knowing* such actions might cause cancer—cigarette smoking and excessive sunbathing excepted.

A while back, a cancer patient named Linda came to her first group meeting at The Wellness Community. Linda had been in a self-help group elsewhere and was told, "Unless you are prepared to accept the blame for the onset of the illness, we can't be of much help to you." Linda believed they were right and had spent several sessions with that group looking for what she had done wrong. "Then," she said, "we found that what I had done was worry too much about my daughter, who, for about six months was thought by her doctors to have multiple sclerosis. I shouldn't have worried so much."

Alice, one of the people in Linda's group, became incensed. "How in heaven's name," asked Alice, "did you come to the conclusion that you did something wrong because you acted as every mother in the world would? When you were worrying, did you know that worry might cause cancer, and if you had known it, would you have stopped worrying about your daughter? That's just silly."

Alice then admitted that she, too, had felt self-blame when she was first diagnosed as having cancer. She told Linda: "I didn't even need a group to help me feel guilty and inadequate. I did it all by myself. You, at least, needed help. When I learned that cancer wasn't my fault, I felt that a massive weight had been taken off my shoulders. The same thing can happen to you. Go back and tell that group they don't know what they're talking about. Tell them nobody except smokers can be to blame for cancer. Ask them what they're doing to make sure they don't get cancer. Tell them if they're so sure the cancer patient must be to blame, they'd better work out a surefire way to ensure that it doesn't happen to them, so they don't have to blame themselves if it does."

When Alice finished, she sat down to ringing applause. We all agreed with her, and when we looked at Linda, she was laughing. She, too, was becoming convinced that self-blame has no place in the cancer patient's life.

The question often asked after a discussion of the possibility of blame for the onset of cancer is: "If I didn't cause the cancer, how can I help to recover from it?" That question is like asking, "Since I didn't cause the weed to grow, how can I kill it?" If you believe that your actions can influence your immune system, which in turn may alter the course of the disease toward health, what difference does it make whether you caused the illness?

Scientists who have made the investigation of psychological aspects of cancer their life's work do not say that you can help cure yourself only if you caused the illness, nor do they say that since you did not cause the cancer, it's futile to even try to help yourself. What they would say if asked is: *"If you fight for recovery, you may enhance the possibility of that recovery, whether or not you were to blame for the development of the disease."*

CHAPTER 32

∼

Know You Are Not to Blame
If the Illness Is Not Progressing
As You Want It To

There is the possibility that some cancer patients who try some of these suggestions, and who are not recovering as quickly as they think they should, might believe that it's their fault—that if they were better at meditation, being partners with their physicians, releasing their anger, or if they had done "it" more often or with more concentration they would be sure to recover. That just isn't so. Recovery is not in your complete control. Biology can overcome psychology.

While there are many ways you can participate in your fight for recovery, and there is the distinct possibility that your activity may have a positive effect on the course of the illness, you don't have the power to ensure recovery. If you believe that recovery is guaranteed if you do it *right*, any setback will be seen as proof of your inadequacy. *But no matter what happens, you are not inadequate. What you are doing is right and proper for you and you are doing it as well as anyone in the world can do it.* And just because there is no assurance of winning, you should not stop trying.

If we refused to enter any race we weren't sure of winning, we would enter precious few races. If we didn't take any job unless we were guaranteed that we would be a great success, most of us would always be out of work. Almost nothing in life is certain, and there are very few situations over which we have complete control. In that respect, the fight for recovery from cancer is not much different from most other efforts we make in life.

For cancer patients, the advice of this chapter is to go for it with all your might, with the full realization that just making the effort makes you a winner. Take credit for the successes, but don't assume any blame if progress is slow. Be aware that there are no failures, because no matter what you have done, you have done all you could, and no one could do it better. You are the best you that ever was or ever will be. Don't forget it!

CHAPTER 33

⌐2⌐

Be Careful of What You Eat

For many years there were those who held that nutrition had no effect on health. Those days are past. Every medical professional I know now believes that what you eat plays a part in maintaining and, perhaps, regaining health. For that reason, learning what one should and should not eat is important to everyone. It is even more important to you as a cancer patient, since in addition to the effect certain foods may have on your physical well-being, there is evidence that there are foods that may exacerbate feelings of distress and others that will make you feel better.

In addition to the physical benefits of being on a specific food regimen, there is a psychological benefit. At least three times every day you are taking back some control of your life by making a conscious decision about what you will and won't eat. Each time you reject a food you believe is unhealthy or eat a food that is "good for you," you are taking back just that much more control—you are participating in your fight for recovery.

Although an extensive review of nutrition and cancer is far beyond the scope of this book, I will set forth, with the help of Carolyn F. Katzin, M.S., some basics to whet your appetite for this subject. In the past several years many of the participants at The Wellness Community in Southern California have come to rely on Carolyn, who has established an enviable reputation as a nutritionist and health educator, particularly in this field. At our request, she prepared *The Wellness Community Nutrition Handbook,* which is

included here as Appendix 3. Several other publications have
addressed themselves to nutrition and cancer. They are *Beating
Cancer with Nutrition* by Patrick Quillin, Ph.D., R.D. (1994), *The
Cancer Recovery Eating Program* by Daniel W. Dixon, M.D. (1994),
and "Eating and Cancer," published by the National Cancer Institute. You can order this last pamphlet by calling 1-(800)-4-
CANCER.

Carolyn has lectured and written extensively on several exciting discoveries having to do with decreasing the risk of developing
cancer by eating certain foods and rejecting others. It can be
extrapolated from each of these that if certain nutritional rules can
reduce the risk of developing cancer, it is reasonable to believe that
they may also have a positive effect on inhibiting the spread and
growth of the illness. As an example, we now have substantial
evidence that the amount of fat and animal protein in the diet
affects the risk of developing certain types of cancer. The experts
tell us that it is best to reduce the total amount of fat intake to
between 15 percent and 30 percent of total intake. You might
consider following that suggestion as part of your fight for recovery. You might also increase your intake of soy protein, which
appears to have a particularly important role to play in the prevention of cancer. Soy is one of the legume family of plants, which
also includes red kidney beans, garbanzo beans, green beans, and
peas.

A third, and equally valuable, food choice would be to include
vegetables from the cruciferous family, such as broccoli, cauliflower, cabbage, and brussels sprouts. These contain plant protective factors that have been shown to be anticarcinogenic in animal
and tissue-culture studies. These are just a few of the ever-growing
lists of foods we have learned are protective. This is a method of
fighting for recovery that I strongly suggest you consider.

I would not feel comfortable unless, before ending this chapter, I referred you to the warning of the American Cancer Society
as stated in the October 1993 issue of *Ca—A Cancer Journal For
Clinicians,* which reads as follows: "After studying the literature
and other available information, the American Cancer Society has

found no evidence that any specific dietary regimen is useful as a cure for cancer. Lacking such evidence, the American Cancer Society strongly urges individuals with cancer not to use dietary programs as an exclusive or primary means of treatment." The thrust of that article is to warn patients not to substitute dietary regimens for conventional medical treatment. I strongly agree.

CHAPTER 34

Exercise

The suggestion in this chapter will be short and direct. Exercise can be an important part in a cancer patient's fight for recovery. In his article "Exercise in the Prevention and Treatment of Cancer," which appeared in a 1993 issue of *Sports Medicine,* Roy J. Shephard of the University of Toronto Medical School, a respected researcher in the area of exercise and health, sums up the benefits of exercise for the cancer patient as follows: "An increase of physical activity stimulates appetite, encourages the conversion of lean tissue, improves functional capacity, slows the clinical course of the disease, sets back the age at death and increases the quality of life. Exercise has an immediate mood-elevating effect and thus can help the cancer patient psychologically. All of these seem good arguments for persuading the cancer patient to involve himself or herself in physical activity." As I said, exercise can be an important part of your fight for recovery.

Although this statement is positive, definite, and specific there are uncertainties as to how long and how vigorous those exercises should be. There is some thought that too much exercise can be counterproductive. Therefore, I cannot stress too strongly the need to discuss the question of exercise with your physician.

CHAPTER 35

Volunteer

The jury is still out on whether volunteering will help in your fight for recovery, but there is that possibility, and it can't do any harm. My personal observation is that those who volunteer seem to be happier than those who don't. It is, of course, common knowledge that volunteering to help others always results in a glow of self-satisfaction and an awareness of the goodness of one's fellow human beings. Also, there is enough scientific information that volunteering may have a positive effect on health that you might consider volunteering as an additional method of fighting for recovery.

In 1990 Howard F. Andrews, Ph.D., conducted a study of the effects volunteering had on physical and mental well-being. In a 1990 issue of *Advances* he reported the results as follows:

> There is no basis in this research for a claim that volunteer activity is a cure-all or provides any guarantee of immunity from major illness. On the other hand, the research of the relationship between health and helping does indicate that those volunteers who help strangers frequently have a very real health advantage over those who do not engage in such helping activity. In summary, the results of this study suggest that volunteer activity, particularly when performed frequently and directed toward strangers, can be added to the growing list

of life-style and social network factors associated with physical and mental well-being.

There are many participants of Wellness Communities throughout the United States who are consistent volunteers, doing everything from talking to new cancer patients to helping with the filing. When asked why they do it, they all say that it's because it makes them feel good—not because it's healthy. That's enough reason for me.

CHAPTER 36

Summation

I spent quite a bit of time asking myself how to write a final chapter to this book, without coming up with an answer and I now know why. There is no final chapter—the fight goes on. The methods you have learned here to fight for your recovery can be used for as long as you like. Those methods of enhancing your immune system are not only useful while you are ill; they can be a part of your life forever. And this book does not have all the answers—there are many methods you will think of to become an even more effective Patient Active.

So this is not the end. My hopes, and those of all the others who have helped write this book, are with you. As I said in the very beginning, like your friends, family, physician, and health care team, above everything else, we want you to recover, and I hope that this book has been helpful. I wish you the best forever, and I hope everything turns out exactly as you want it to. Good luck!

IV

QUESTIONS CANCER PATIENTS ASK

QUESTION 1

∽

Are the Methods Suggested an Alternative to Conventional Medical Treatment?

The answer to that question is a resounding "NO." The Patient Active concept, the suggestions made here, and all aspects of The Wellness Community are in support of and adjunctive to conventional medical treatment. One way of describing the Patient Active concept is that it combines the will of the patient with the skill of the physicians—a powerful combination. We are proud that over 350 physicians are members of the Professional Advisory Boards of Wellness Communities throughout the United States. You can be sure that those physicians would not be involved with us, or endorse the Patient Active concept, if we were an alternative to conventional medical treatment. Truth to tell, I wouldn't be involved with an organization or concept that was not in support of conventional medical treatment.

Just a few years ago, the type of patient involvement suggested here was considered by many as a useless waste of time and, to some, downright injurious. That's no longer true. I have yet to meet a physician who does not believe that patient involvement as a partner in the fight for recovery is a step in the right direction. As Richard Steckel, M.D., Director of the Johnson Comprehensive Cancer Center, UCLA, said in the preface to the first edition of this book, "I have yet to meet a physician who would not prefer to relate to his or her cancer patient as a partner in the fight for recovery." It is my experience that Dr. Steckel was speaking for most if not all physicians.

Support of the Patient Active concept by physicians is also indicated by the following statements made by several oncologists. Since the methods described in this book were all originated and tested at and are now being used at The Wellness Community, the following observations about that program are actually observations about the methods suggested in this book.

Peter Kennedy, M.D., a medical oncologist in Pasadena, said: "When patients enter The Wellness Community they are more assertive. They often tolerate therapy better. They're more willing to do what must be done to fight the disease. As an oncologist, I spend less time fighting fear and more time fighting cancer and pressing rehabilitative efforts. I win and my patients win. Good for Wellness."

Rebecca Bechhold, M.D., an oncologist at Bethesda North Hospital in Cincinnati, observed: "Obviously, my patients [who are Patients Active] call with their medical questions, but they don't feel the need to call about every little thing. Their anxiety level drops. They feel more confident and they're able to handle things better."

Robert Lowitz, M.D., Director of Oncology, John Muir Medical Center, Walnut Creek, California, when talking to a group of physicians about The Wellness Community, said: "What I see as a provider, when the patients come [to me] following their weekly visits [to The Wellness Community], is that the somatic symptoms of the patient are lessened, their anxiety level is lessened, their depression is lessened and their energy is up and they're better. I'm not sure they live longer, but I know they live better."

Hundreds of physicians demonstrate their belief in the proposition that the cancer patient's mental and perhaps physical well-being may benefit from participation in the fight for recovery by referring their patients to The Wellness Community. The names of those physicians who are members of the Professional Advisory Board of The Wellness Community—National are listed in the front of this book. I believe you will agree that it's a rather impressive list.

WILL MY PHYSICIAN APPROVE
OF MY PARTICIPATION IN THE FIGHT
FOR RECOVERY?

I believe that all of the above information is a significant indication
that your physician and health care team will not only approve of
but encourage such participation. What more is there to say?

*When I first came to The Wellness Community, I was very sick—mostly,
it seemed to me, from the chemotherapy I was receiving from my doctor. I
had decided that enough was enough—I had had it. No more chemo and
no more doctor for me. When I became a part of a Wellness Community
group of eleven other people with cancer, and made my announcement, they
looked at me as if I were crazy. And that's what they said: "Are you crazy?
That's the way to fight for recovery." And they told me story after story of
how their treatment had made all the difference for them. I followed their
advice. I have now been in remission for over thirteen months and I'm sure
that I wouldn't be here if it were not for the chemo and the combined efforts
of my doctor and me. My doctor now sends all of his patients to The
Wellness Community.*

Leonard

QUESTION 2

⌒♈︎

Do Cancer Patients Who Participate in Support Groups Abandon Conventional Medical Treatment?

No! Two studies give credence to that answer. The first, a survey at two Wellness Community facilities in 1989, under the guidance of Michael Goldstein, Ph.D., of the UCLA School of Public Health, revealed that of the ninety-four participants surveyed *all* were under the care of conventional physicians when they entered the program; they had been in The Wellness Community an average of fourteen and a half months, and at the time of the survey, all but six were still under conventional medical care. Of those six, two were in complete remission and no longer needed a physician, two had had arguments with their physicians, and two didn't answer the question. That puts to rest, once and for all, two assumptions that have concerned the medical profession for some time: that cancer patients use psychosocial efforts as an alternative to conventional medical treatment, and that those who become active participants in their fight for recovery abandon conventional medicine. It just doesn't happen.

Another study that substantiates the concept that those who participate in complementary medicine do not abandon conventional medical care was reported under the title "Unconventional Medicine in the United States," by Dr. E. M. Eisenberg, reported in the *New England Journal of Medicine* in 1993.

That study investigated the use of alternative medicine in the United States by telephone interviews of 1,537 subjects. The key conclusion of that study was that "no respondent in this study who identified cancer as a principal medical problem reported seeing a provider of alternative therapy *without also seeing a medical doctor for the condition.*" (Emphasis added.) I believe that answers the question.

What Is Cancer?

To outline, cancer occurs when (1) an abnormal cell appears in the body, (2) continues to divide and subdivide after it should have stopped, and (3) eventually forms a clump of cells, called a tumor, which (4) if unchecked will grow large enough to interfere with the delivery of nutrients and oxygen to nearby organs; (5) the abnormal cells are of the type that can survive in parts of the body other than where they originated. These cells are called cancer cells.

To explain in more detail, the human body is a collection of cells that perform separate, specific functions, each linked to the others and operating in a highly regulated manner. In a normal cycle, a cell is born, matures and performs its designated function, and then "dies." When a cell dies it must be replaced by a new cell, and this is accomplished by a nearby cell dividing in two and then those two dividing again and so on until the exact number of required new cells is achieved. Under normal circumstances, the birth and death of a cell is an exquisitely precise process. But problems arise when, for reasons still unknown, a normal cell divides to replace other cells and gives birth to an abnormal cell that does not stop dividing when it is supposed to and refuses to die on schedule. Such cells if unchecked divide and subdivide without end and eventually join together to form a tumor. As the tumor becomes larger, it impedes the functioning of nearby organs by intruding on their space and interfering with their supply of oxygen and nutrients. Eventually, unless the growth is stopped or the tumor removed the healthy organs are destroyed.

There are two types of abnormal cells. The first type of abnormal cell can survive only at its place of origin. That type of abnormal cell forms a tumor where it originates. This is called a benign tumor, which, while serious, can often be surgically removed, thereby ending the problem. The other type of abnormal cell is more dangerous because not only won't it stop divid-. ing when it's supposed to but also it can thrive anyplace in the body. The ability to travel and survive in areas other than the primary site is called metastasis. That type of cell is a cancer cell. Cancer cells form a tumor at the primary site and at places to which it metastasizes. That's cancer—the generic name for over a hundred diseases that share the general characteristics of malignant cells. For cancer to be successfully treated, not only must the original tumor be dealt with but the spread (metastasis) must be stopped.

The next important aspect of cancer is that we all have cancer cells proliferating in our bodies some of the time and the reason we all don't develop cancer is that our immune systems, as described next, are strong enough to destroy the cancer cells when they appear. Motion pictures have actually shown cancer cells being attacked and destroyed by the cells of the immune system. It's an inspiring sight. Some cancer patients cheer when they see it.

THE IMMUNE SYSTEM:
OUR FIRST LINE OF DEFENSE

Our immune system is an intricate system designed to protect the body from disease and from "foreigners" that invade through a break in the skin, via food or other ingested matter, or by way of the air we breathe or the rays to which we are exposed. For cancer to take hold, the cancer cell must appear and the immune system must not be strong enough to rid the body of that cancer cell. One way to think about cancer is not that the cancer cell is strong but that the body's immune system is not strong enough to carry out its assigned function of removing cancer cells from the body. This view of cancer is generally known as the immune surveillance theory.

QUESTION 4

What Causes Cancer?

We know from the answer to the previous question that for cancer to occur two events must take place simultaneously: (1) A cancer cell must appear and (2) the body's immune system is too weak to destroy it. That raises the following two questions: First, what causes a cancer cell to appear, and second, what factors determine how strong the immune system is? To answer those questions, we must first look at the three elements that affect both the production of cells and the strength of the immune system. They are (1) genetics—the body we inherit, (2) environment—the world in which we live, and (3) behavior—the ways we react to life events.

Genetics. Those are the physical characteristics we have inherited. They determine the strength of our immune systems and the number of cancer cells we produce. We have no control over this aspect of our lives.

Environment. This includes the air we breath, the food we eat, the liquids we drink, the cigarettes we smoke and generally, the physical circumstances in which we live. We have only limited control over this aspect of our lives even if we are ever so careful. It is well established that an environment high in substances such as cigarette smoke, asbestos, or certain foods, all of which are called carcinogens, can cause a substantial increase in the number of cancer cells produced.

To illustrate the role played by the environment, assume that John has inherited an immune system strong enough to deal with the cancer cells his body produces under normal circumstances. Then, assume further, that John takes up smoking or gets a job in an asbestos factory which increase the number of cancer cells he produces. It is quite possible that his immune system, strong enough to protect him under normal circumstances, may not be robust enough to protect him from the additional cancer cells that now appear in his body. Thus, you see that environmental factors can play a significant part in the onset of the illness. There is no evidence that the environment has any effect on the strength of the immune system.

Behavior encompasses the way we live our lives and react to life events. As you will see, our behavior and emotions can affect the strength of our immune systems. Since the strength of our immune systems may affect the course of the illness and since behavior may affect the strength of our immune systems, and since we have some control over our behavior, it follows that we may have some control over the course of the illness. That's the point—we may have some control over the course of the illness. There is no evidence that behavior has any affect on the production of cancer cells.

It's important to notice at this point that the immune system we inherited can be so strong that no matter how many cancer cells we produce or what our environment or behavior is, we will not develop cancer. It could also be so weak that cancer may be our lot even if we live the most pristine of lives and produce very few cancer cells.

OUTLINE OF FACTORS AFFECTING THE ONSET OF CANCER

	GENETICS	ENVIRONMENT	BEHAVIOR
PRODUCTION OF CANCER CELLS	Controlling	Can affect production of cancer cells	No evidence of any influence on production of cancer cells
STRENGTH OF THE IMMUNE SYSTEM	Controlling	No evidence of any influence on strength of immune system	Can affect strength of immune system
OUR CONTROL OVER THESE FACTORS	None	Very little	More than very little

HOW OUR BEHAVIOR AFFECTS THE STRENGTH OF OUR IMMUNE SYSTEMS

To understand how our behavior affects our immune system we must first understand the fight-or-flight response. You will see how descriptive that phrase is as you read along.

FIGHT-OR-FLIGHT RESPONSE

A cave man is walking down a trail when he senses that there is a tiger in the bush. He now has two choices—he can continue and fight the tiger or he can run away. In either event, evolution, in order to assure the survival of the species, has provided certain automatic physical responses—the production of certain chemicals by the brain which makes the one in danger able to fight more fiercely or run away more quickly—the fight-or-flight response. You may have noticed this reaction with your own experience with a frightening experience—an increased heart rate and respiration and an alertness you don't usually have. We share the fight-or-flight response with every mammal on earth.

This fight-or-flight response creates a problem for modern man for three reasons: (1) The chemicals produced by the brain in response to fear depress the immune system, (2) the fight-or-flight response is not only evoked by fear of physical injury, it is also triggered by any and all unpleasant emotions such as sadness, hurt feelings, or anxiety, and (3) the fight-or-flight reaction evoked by an emotional response to a life event can last for a very long time.

This is important because if the depressed immune system lasts for only a short period of time, it is unlikely that a cancer cell will appear at that exact moment. But if the condition lasts for an extended period of time—weeks, months, or years—it is more likely that a cancer cell will appear while the depressed immune system is too weak to handle it.

That was no problem in the early days of human evolution because all threats were resolved in one way or another in a short period of time, and when the danger was past, the brain stopped producing the immune-depressing chemicals and the immune system returned to its normal strength. But, in these more civilized times, anxiety can last for weeks, months, or a lifetime, and I repeat for emphasis: during this extended period of time while the brain is still producing chemicals that depress the immune system, it is more likely that the cancer cell will appear while the immune system is not strong enough to handle it.

What is more important to you as a cancer patient is that if cancer is already present and you are reacting to life events in ways that trigger the immune-depressing fight-or-flight response, your immune system may not be as strong as it would be if your emotional responses to life events were such that the brain was not reacting as if there was a tiger in the bush. This book is all about ways to avoid the "fight or flight" response and thereby strengthen your immune system.

QUESTION 5

ℭ⁀

How Can Your Efforts Enhance the Possibility of Recovery?

We have learned from the answers to the previous questions and the anecdote of the transplanted kidney told in Chapter One that even after cancer has been diagnosed, if the immune system becomes stronger it may be able to rid the body of that cancer. That's exactly what physicians seek to do when they introduce immune enhancers such as interferon or interleukin-2 into the body—strengthen the immune system so that, hopefully, it will be strong enough to destroy the tumor.

The methods suggested in this book are for the purpose of accomplishing that very result—strengthening the immune system—by psychological means. The possibility that psychological methods may accomplish the desired result is given credence by the discoveries of Psychoneuroimmunology (PNI). Those findings suggest that pleasant emotions enhance the immune system and long-term, unremitting unpleasant emotions depress the immune system. They also suggest that the more intense the emotion and the longer it lasts the greater its effect on our immune systems. The purpose of the suggestions made here is to make available to cancer patients the tools to maximize pleasant emotions and minimize unpleasant emotions, in the hope that the immune system will become strong enough to alter the course of the disease toward health.

The first step in this line of thinking is that our coping style—our behavior—determines, to some extent, the stress we undergo and the amplitude and duration of that stress. It follows, then, that if we control our reactions to traumatic events or confine them to a limited period of time, we may significantly enhance the possibility of recovery. This observation can be thought about in the following form:

- The strength of our immune systems affects the course of the illness—the stronger the immune system the more likely the recovery.
- Long-term, unremitting stress depresses our immune systems.
- The less intense the stress and the less time it continues the less the suppression of the immune system.
- Pleasant emotions enhance our immune systems.
- The more intense the pleasant emotions and the longer they continue the more the immune system is strengthened.
- We have some control over the amplitude and duration of stress.
- Therefore, we may have some control over the course of the illness.

Assume this time that John has worked for ten years in an asbestos factory (an environmental factor), where his immune system (an inherited factor) has been sufficiently robust to prevent the development of cancer. However, if John's wife leaves him and his children become delinquent, and if he reacts violently to these events over a long time, that reaction to the situation may suppress his immune system so that it is unable to destroy all the cancer cells as they appear.

Notice that it is not the stressors that suppress his immune system; it is John's *reaction* to those stressors that does the damage.

There is also Robert, who has cancer. Before he had cancer, he had a partner in business who was not working as hard as Robert thought he should. It was a source of great stress to Robert. Robert is also the type of person who becomes angry over life events, such as being cut off in traffic. Robert learned that his constant stress is depressing his immune system and that if he reduced that stress his immune system might become strong enough to have a positive effect on the course of the illness. He also learned that he has some control over how he reacts to those situations. It's now up to Robert. Robert can work on this issue by using some or all of the suggestions in this book. So can you.

QUESTION 6

What Is The Wellness Community?

Since I have constantly referred to The Wellness Community as the source of the information and suggestions offered here, I thought you might want to know what that organization is and what it does. Also, if there is one of our facilities in your area, you might want to find out how it can be helpful to you. The following statements about the Community will set the stage for further discussion.

- All the services provided by The Wellness Community are free. We don't charge for anything under any circumstances. A list of these services is set forth in Appendix 1.
- The Wellness Community is a nonresidential program where people with cancer come to learn whatever they need to know to fight for their recovery using psychological methods as an adjunct to conventional medical care. It is not a hospice or a place where cancer patients learn to die or adapt their lives to cancer.
- The hope of everyone associated with The Wellness Community is that as many cancer patients as possible recover to the greatest extent possible. We have many wonderful stories to tell about recoveries and remissions. Of course, not everyone who comes to The Wellness Community recovers from the illness, but many do. We take no credit for those recoveries, but are delighted when they happen.

- In each Wellness Community throughout the United States, we have a homelike facility devoted solely to our program.
- All facilitators at The Wellness Community are licensed psychotherapists and are specially trained in The Wellness Community's unique methods under the tutelage of the faculty of the National Training Center in Santa Monica, California.
- Each of our methods is based on scientific fact or reasonable scientific hypothesis.
- The Wellness Community has thirteen facilities nationwide and six facilities in development. We will have facilities in fifty cities by the year 2000. Information about The Wellness Communities throughout the United States is included in Appendix 5.
- At the time of this writing, we have psychosocially supported over 30,000 participants and provide such support to over 3,500 each week.
- The Wellness Community has a parallel program for family members of cancer patients.
- The following statement is the basic concept which, since day one, has been the foundation on which The Wellness Community and the Patient Active concept are built:

Cancer patients who participate in their fight for recovery along with their physicians and other health care professionals will improve the quality of their lives and may enhance the possibility of their recovery.

I am proud of that statement, made originally in 1982, because studies reported in scientific journals in the early 1990s have proven true what we have surmised for so long.

HISTORY

In the first half of the twentieth century, medical science uncovered some of the secrets about cancer, resulting in new medical treatments such as chemotherapy, surgery, and radiation therapy. It was also during this period that more sophisticated diagnostic procedures were defined. Then, either because of earlier diagnosis or as a result of improved treatment, cancer patients began to live longer. It was soon observed that the cancer patients who were living with cancer for an extended period of time were exhibiting symptoms of extreme psychological distress of a nature not usually experienced in other diseases.

Then, in a parallel series of events, scientists such as Walter B. Cannon and Hans Selye discovered that there is a direct link between the workings of the mind and the physical condition of the body. Based upon that foundation, research in the 1970s by scientists Robert Ader and Nicholas Cohen uncovered additional facts about the connection between the mind and the body and formalized the study of that link, which was called psychoneuro-immunology—PNI for short. The popular press now calls it "the mind/body connection." The long word, however, is quite useful. It describes the question originally asked by the scientists in this field: Do emotions (psycho) transmitted by the nervous system (neuro) have an effect on the immune system (immunology), which is the body's first line of defense against cancer and other diseases? In short, do emotions have an effect on physical well-being? Within a relatively short time those scientists found their answer—a resounding "yes": our emotions have a direct effect on our physical well-being. That was a turning point in the history of medicine. Since then, and continuing to the present, the scientists working in this field have been seeking to determine *exactly* what effect emotions have on the immune system and physical well-being. As you will discover, the progress in PNI over the past twenty years has been extraordinary.

In the 1960s and 1970s, another new area of investigation

emerged—to determine the most efficient methods by which the findings of PNI can be used to help well people avoid illness and ill people, particularly people with cancer, recover from illness. That latter area, often called psycho-oncology, is of course the area of most interest to you and to all of us who have spent the last decade and a half doing theoretical and practical research in the field. That was the fertile ground that existed when I became involved with the "science" of the psychological aspects of cancer therapy.

I came to that science through a rather circuitous route. For thirty years (from 1950 to 1980) I practiced law in New York City and Beverly Hills, and for some of those years (1966 to 1975) I participated in and studied an organization that used a combination of communal living and psychotherapeutic methods—groups—to support people fighting for recovery from substance abuse. I believe it was the first "therapeutic community" devoted to the relief of a psychological problem—addiction to drugs. It was there I became aware of the tremendous power for psychological good that can come from a therapeutic community—how healthy such a community can be for someone with a serious illness.

In 1972 when my wife, Harriet, had a bilateral mastectomy, our friends at the community didn't treat her as a second-class citizen because she had cancer. Our friends there didn't look upon her as "dying." To them, she was the same Harriet Benjamin she had been before the operation, except she had cancer. She encountered none of the rejection so many cancer patients face daily. She had all her friends beside her, supporting her fight to regain her health. She received love, support, and encouragement but experienced no knee-jerk sympathy, no pity, no reluctance to be with her because of the illness.

There is no doubt in my mind that all of this support improved the quality of Harriet's life. I also can't help but believe that it had something to do with the fact that since her mastectomy, Harriet has been leading a very active, symptom-free life. This experience had a deep and lasting effect on me. On reflection, I know that it was then that I learned, on some subconscious level, that camaraderie, togetherness, and support have a beneficial effect on people with serious illness. And when I later became familiar with the problems of cancer patients, this knowledge surfaced and gave rise to The Wellness Community concept of the Patient Active.

In 1976, while continuing to practice law, I became active in an organization that was created to train psychologists to treat individuals with life-threatening illnesses. For the next five years, I spent all my free time studying the psychosocial aspects of serious illness and interacting with a great many cancer patients. It was there that I observed that cancer patients have a tremendous need for support, hope, encouragement, and involvement in the fight for recovery; that they have become the modern-day lepers; and that most cancer patients are, to one extent or another, abandoned both physically and emotionally by their family and friends, just when they need support the most. I learned, both in the world of academia and by interacting with a great many cancer patients, that in addition to financial problems and fear of suffering and death, the three most debilitating psychosocial problems that accompany cancer are feelings of helplessness and hopelessness, unwanted aloneness, and loss of control. I also learned that life does not end with the diagnosis of cancer and that there is always room for hope, joy, and involvement in life while fighting for recovery; that negative emotions can have negative physical effects and that positive emotions may be physically beneficial; that togetherness is good for people and unwanted aloneness can be physically harmful; and that there has been a wealth of material published over the past twenty years indicating strongly that an individual's efforts in the fight for recovery may enhance the possibility of recovery. Somehow, that knowledge filled me with joy and hope.

In 1981, quite suddenly and without any effort on my part, all I had learned about the benefits of community, my understanding of the mind/body connection (PNI), and my knowledge of the positive results that flow from psychotherapeutic interchange between cancer patients merged and gave birth to the Patient Active concept, *a series of psychological and emotional guidelines cancer patients can use in their fight for recovery.* Immediately thereafter I knew that I would start a program to make the concept available to all cancer patients—The Wellness Community. I didn't know how, but I knew I would.

Frankly, I was awed by the breadth and potential of the concept, and I became anxious when I realized, after investigation, that there was no program based on the same or similar concept, that one had to be started, and that I was the one to do it. How was I to do that? Should I, a lawyer with a very active practice, give all that up? Did I have the courage? Without trying to answer any of those questions I started to work on getting the ideas down on paper. Out flowed the basic outline of the concept, the design of the program, the methods we would use to overcome specific problems, the procedures we would use to teach the concept to licensed therapists, and all the other techniques we would use to support cancer patients in their fight for recovery. Interestingly, although the program is constantly evolving and growing, the methods and techniques I used in those early days remain, in large part—with a great deal of honing and refinement—the methods and techniques we use today.

It was then I went to see Norman Cousins. He loved the idea. He encouraged me to give it a try. He was the only one. I thought about nothing else for about six months and then, once again quite suddenly, in December 1981, almost without any thought, I told my law partner that I was retiring from the law to devote my full time to opening and administering The Wellness Community. I would be less than candid if I did not report that he and all my friends thought I was crazy. However, on January 1, 1982, I quit, and had nothing to do but start The Wellness Community. I was then joined by Shannon Behrens, now Shannon McGowan, a licensed therapist and former cervical cancer patient who believed in the concept and was willing to be part of a project as untested as this one.

Getting The Wellness Community off the ground was not always easy. However, one problem about which I had been warned by all my friends did not materialize. From the day I started to discuss the project I was told that the medical profession would "shoot the project out of the sky." That's not what happened at all. The medical community acted in exactly the way I hope I would have acted under those circumstances. They watched with skepticism for the first six months, and then when they determined that we were not going to charge, that we did not believe that we had the answer to cancer, and that we considered our program as an adjunct to conventional medical treatment and not an alternative, they wholeheartedly supported our work.

The first action we took was to find a little yellow house in Santa Monica, California, much in need of renovation and refurbishing. While working to renovate that house I drafted and redrafted the brochures describing the services we were planning to offer. That wasn't an easy job. I had no model to look to. However, I was sure of what we were going to do. I just didn't know how to say it so that everyone would understand it. Don't forget, in 1982 the entire field of PNI was known to few physicians and even fewer laymen, and to almost everyone the thought of using psychological techniques to battle a physical illness was considered, at the very least, esoteric. As far as psycho-oncology was concerned, you can count on your fingers and toes the number of people who were knowledgeable about that field, and certainly, a psychotherapeutic community for cancer patients had never been tried. I was on my own. To describe The Wellness Community I had to start from scratch and make up the words.

However, after about six months the little yellow house was ready and the brochures were finished. It was then we realized with a shock that we had no participants and we didn't know where or how to get them. But by a series of coincidences, we came into contact with a group of cancer patients and offered them our services, and six came to our opening on June 15, 1982. We were off and running. As I look back on our beginning stages, I am amazed at our courage.

When I mention coincidences I feel obliged to say that there have been more of those "accidentally happening events" than you can imagine. Every time I was at an impasse or faced with a problem I didn't know how to solve or needed someone special to help me over a particular hurdle, what I needed seemed to appear. For all of that, I am very grateful.

I would also like to say a few words about Norman Cousins. Not only was he the only one to encourage me to "go for it"; after we opened, he was always there when we needed him. He became Honorary Chair of our Board and his fame and credibility made many of the paths we had to travel easier than they would have been without him. For that, too, I am grateful.

Our program was a success from the start. Shannon did the first group and she and I provided all the rest of the program and we started to grow. Our growth is indicated by the description of our facilities nationwide (Appendix 5), the more than 350 physicians who are on our Professional Advisory Boards, and the hundreds and hundreds of physicians who send their patients to us. I cannot tell you how proud I am to be on the same team with all of them.

One question that always comes up is, where did the money come from? For the first two years Harriet and I paid for everything. After that, we looked to those charitable people, businesses, and foundations who wanted to help cancer patients fight for recovery. That's where the money comes from.

APPENDICES

APPENDIX 1

_cᴗ__

Services Provided by
The Wellness Community

(Always Without Charge)

The Wellness Community is, above everything else, a community—a place where people with cancer and their families can be with others to build support and a sense of extended family to mitigate feelings of unwanted aloneness. It is a place where they can come to learn whatever it is they need to know, on the psychological and emotional level, to fight for recovery along with their medical team. Every aspect of The Wellness Community free program listed below is designed to help patients fight for recovery and improve the quality of their lives.

1. **Homelike Facility Available All Day:** The Wellness Community provides a comfortable and homelike facility where cancer patients and their families can participate in any of the numerous activities offered. They meet with others to learn to involve themselves in the fight to get well and get on with life despite cancer. All of our participants are invited, encouraged, and welcomed to use the facilities in much the same way as those of a community or neighborhood center. Participants and staff are present throughout the day and evening as well as on weekends.

2. **Orientation Meetings:** At these twice-a-week, informal drop-in groups led by people who have or have had cancer, cancer patients new to The Wellness Community meet others similarly situated. Here they learn that the diagnosis is not always a sentence of death, that life does not end with the

diagnosis, that they can participate in their fight for recovery along with their physicians, and that there is hope—always hope. It is at these meetings that they get an overview of the services they can use.

3. **Participant Groups:** These are ongoing two-hour weekly groups led by licensed psychotherapists who are specially trained in dealing with the problems of cancer patients, where participants (1) become part of an extended family of those who understand, (2) learn new and different methods for dealing with the physical and emotional problems associated with the illness, and (3) perhaps relieve some of the stress in their lives. This is for the participant who is actively fighting for physical recovery and wants to make a weekly commitment to the same group. After a participant is asymptomatic for eighteen months, his or her involvement can continue in a variety of ways such as the Wellness Connection, the alumni registry, the speakers' bureau, parties, and workshops.

4. **Family Groups:** At these two-hour weekly support groups, led by licensed psychotherapists who are specially trained in dealing with the problems of cancer patients, significant others of cancer patients in a Participant Group learn how best to support the person with cancer—much to the benefit of both.

5. **Short-term Individual or Family Counseling:** Six sessions of counseling are provided for individuals or families in crisis, with the emphasis on bringing material back to the group. These are done by professionals in training or licensed interns at The Wellness Community. Requests are made through the facilitator of the ongoing group, and scheduling depends upon the availability of the interns.

6. **Visualization/relaxation:** Each week, there are sessions where participants are taught by example how to involve themselves in the self-help type of procedure suggested by Herbert

Benson, M.D., in his book *The Relaxation Response* and by O. Carl Simonton, M.D., in his book *Getting Well Again*. The combination of the two methods is described by Harold H. Benjamin, Ph.D., in his book *From Victim to Victor*. These methods are used by many hospitals and physicians to help cancer patients alleviate the effects of stress.

7. **Education:** Several times each month, lectures and dialogues are presented by authorities in fields of interest to cancer patients, such as oncologists, psychologists, insurance specialists, and attorneys knowledgeable about the rights of cancer patients. Of course, The Wellness Community takes no advocacy position. Attendance is on a drop-in basis.

8. **Workshops:** Also several times each month, there are workshops presented by experts in matters such as nutrition, biofeedback, moderate exercise, art therapy, and journal writing. Attendance is on a drop-in basis.

9. **Special Groups for Specific Types of Cancer:** Special groups are presented on an ongoing basis which consider specific areas of concern to cancer patients, such as breast, prostate, and ovarian cancer networking.

10. **Wellness Connection:** In this twice-a-month drop-in group, participants of The Wellness Community who have "graduated" from Participant Groups come together for support and to share with other cancer patients the specific expertise earned only by having been a cancer patient.

11. **Community Events:** Social gatherings such as seasonal parties, potlucks, charade nights, Joke Fests, sing-alongs, and other events bring participants together to laugh and play.

‹շ—

The Wellness Community Patient/Oncologist Statement

Drafted by Oncologists Richard Steckel, Michael Van Scoy Mosher, Laurence Heifetz, and Fred P. Rosenfelt

The effective treatment of serious illness requires a considerable effort by both the patient and the physician. A clear understanding by both of us as to what each of us can realistically and reasonably expect of the other will do much to enhance the outlook. I am giving this "statement" to you as one step in making our relationship as effective and productive as possible. It might be helpful if you would read this statement and, if you think it appropriate, discuss it with me. *As your physician I will make every effort to:*

1. Provide you with the care most likely to be beneficial to you.

2. Inform and educate you about your situation, and the various treatment alternatives. How detailed an explanation is given will be dependent upon your specific desires.

3. Encourage you to ask questions about your illness and its treatment, and answer your questions as clearly as possible. I will also attempt to answer the questions asked by your family; however, my primary responsibility is to you, and I will discuss your medical situation only with those people authorized by you.

4. Remain aware that all major decisions about the course of your care will be made by you. However, I will accept the responsibility for making certain decisions if you want me to.

5. Assist you to obtain other professional opinions if you desire, or if I believe it to be in your best interest.

6. Relate to you as one competent adult to another, always attempting to consider your emotional, social, and psychological needs as well as your physical needs.

7. Spend a reasonable amount of time with you on each return visit unless required by something urgent to do otherwise, and give you my undivided attention during that time.

8. Honor all appointment times unless required by something urgent to do otherwise.

9. Return phone calls as promptly as possible, especially those you indicate are urgent.

10. Make test results available promptly if you desire such reports.

11. Provide you with any information you request concerning my professional training, experience, philosophy, and fees.

12. Respect your desire to try treatment that might not be conventionally accepted. However, I will give you my honest opinion about such unconventional treatments.

13. Maintain my active support and attention throughout the course of the illness.

I hope that you as the patient will make every effort to:

1. Comply with our agreed-upon treatment plan.

2. Be as candid as possible with me about what you need and expect from me.

3. Inform me if you desire another professional opinion.

4. Inform me of all forms of therapy you are involved with.

5. Honor all appointment times unless required by something urgent to do otherwise.

6. Be as considerate as possible of my need to adhere to a schedule to see other patients.

7. Make all phone calls to me during the working hours. Call on nights and weekends only when absolutely necessary.

8. Coordinate the requests of your family and confidants, so that I do not have to answer the same questions about you to several different persons.

APPENDIX 3

౨

The Wellness Community Nutrition Handbook

CONTENTS

INTRODUCTION: CAROLYN KATZIN, M.S., NUTRITIONIST TO THE WELLNESS COMMUNITY NATIONAL TRAINING CENTER

I have had the privilege of counseling participants at The Wellness Community National Training Center since 1986 when we were in the little yellow house in Santa Monica. During this time I have learned more than I have taught. In the following pages I will share with you some of the things I have learned. It would be impossible to write it all down. This summary handbook is a forerunner of a longer book that I am compiling, and if you have any comments or suggestions, I would love to hear from you.

For those of you who are interested in my background, I have a Bachelor of Science degree in nutrition and physiology from London University in my native Britain. I came to California in 1984 to study for my doctorate at UCLA in the field of nutritional science. In 1985 I met my husband, David, who is a holistically oriented physician and scientist. I began counseling his patients, and one of them, Louise Munch, introduced me to The Wellness Community. I graduated from UCLA's School of Public Health with a Master's degree in science, having decided that working with people was more enjoyable for me than research. I maintain an active interest in nutritional research and I work with my husband, who is chairman of the medical and scientific advisory board of an international nutritional-supplement company. I am chair of the nutrition subcommittee for the Coastal Cities Unit of the American Cancer Society and enjoy speaking to both professional and public groups about nutrition and its relationship to health.

STAGES OF CANCER NUTRITION

PREVENTIVE NUTRITION:

- Less than 20% total calories from fat (less than ⅓ from animal sources, e.g., meat, butter).
- High in starch (complex carbohydrates), e.g., beans, pasta, bread, and root vegetables. Low in simple sugars, e.g., candy, desserts.
- Reasonable in protein, i.e., 3–4 oz. servings of lean meat, poultry, or larger, 6–8 oz. servings of mixed beans and rice at lunch and dinner.
- Plenty of antioxidants and botanical factors, found in whole grains, vegetables, and many fruits; e.g., beta carotene, vitamins C and E.
- Moderate quantities overall.
- Wide variety of foods, especially seasonal fruits and vegetables.

DURING TREATMENT:

- Sufficient small, frequent meals that body weight is maintained.
- A little more protein, e.g., more egg whites, fish, and poultry.
- Few dairy products due to possible lactose intolerance which may develop, with abdominal discomfort and diarrhea as symptoms. Live-culture yogurt and hard cheese okay.
- Avoid gas-producing foods such as incompletely cooked beans, excessive amounts of the cabbage family, melons.
- Avoid highly spiced foods.

REGENERATING NUTRITION:

- As for preventive nutrition above, but with special focus on the nutrients needed for regenerating the immune system, e.g., beta carotene, the B vitamins, C, E, selenium, and zinc. Some of these are found in wheat germ—add 1 T to morning cereal.

- At least 5 servings of fruits and vegetables each day.
- Reintroduce dairy products slowly.
- Include antioxidant formula in daily vitamin and mineral supplement.

NUTRITION AND CANCER—GUIDELINES

It is estimated by the National Cancer Institute that at least 35% of all cancers have a nutritional cause. For women this is as high as *one half* of all cancers (breast being particularly related to a high-fat, low-fiber diet). Nutrition is vital for a healthy immune system, which protects us from and provides resistance to cancer. Here is a summary of the American Cancer Society's nutritional guidelines:

1. *Maintain a desirable body weight.* Avoid obesity, which is strongly associated with breast and colorectal cancers. Other cancers shown to be associated with obesity include uterine, gallbladder, kidney, and stomach.

2. *Eat a varied diet.* Variety and moderation are advised.

3. *Include a variety of both vegetables and fruits in your daily diet.* Many studies show a decreased risk of lung, prostate, bladder, esophagus, and stomach cancers with daily fruits and vegetables in the diet. Five servings each day are recommended.

4. *Eat more high-fiber foods, such as whole-grain cereals, legumes, vegetables, and fruits.* Population studies indicate that a high-fiber diet protects against colon cancer. These foods are

wholesome low-calorie substitutes for high-calorie fatty foods.

5. *Cut down on total fat intake.* The average U.S. diet contains about 40% of its calories from fat. A.C.S. recommends reducing to less than 30%. Many people feel that less than 25% is healthier still. No infant or child under two years should be on a low-fat diet, as they require cholesterol for brain development. Exercise is also important in weight maintenance.

6. *Limit consumption of alcoholic beverages, if you drink at all.* Cancer of the oral cavity, larynx, and esophagus is more prevalent in heavy drinkers, especially if they smoke, too. Regular alcohol consumption may also be related to breast cancer in women.

7. *Limit consumption of salt-cured, smoked, and nitrite-preserved foods.* Sausages, fish, hams, and other cured foods may contain carcinogenic tars. Charcoal grilling also produces similar tars, which increase the risk of stomach and esophageal cancers. Nitrosamines are carcinogens which may form from nitrate- and nitrite-cured foods.

Remember—moderation and variety in your diet. Keep active and maintain a healthy weight. Be happy!

NUTRITION DURING TREATMENT

If you have been diagnosed with cancer, one of the most important things for you to consider as part of your whole treatment regimen is nutrition. Eating a healthy diet can make a big difference in the success of your treatment. One simple rule of thumb is to maintain a steady body weight throughout treatment as much as possible. This means neither gaining too much weight nor losing too much (fluctuations of more than, say, 5 lbs. per week).

BEFORE TREATMENT:

Surgery   Eat low-fat, high-protein diet the day before
                  surgery. Supplement with a broad-spectrum
                  multivitamin and -mineral with 100% RDA.
                  Additionally, 500 mg. vitamin C with bio-
                  flavonoids every 8 hours may be beneficial to
                  healing. Stop vitamin E, vitamin K, evening
                  primrose, borage or fish oils supplements 1 week
                  before surgery, as these can cause thinning of the
                  blood.

Radiation   No special diet.

Chemotherapy   Eat low-fat, high-carbohydrate diet the day be-
                  fore chemo. Supplement with multivitamin and
                  -mineral giving 100% RDA.

DURING TREATMENT:

Surgery   As per surgeon's protocol.

Radiation   Extra carbohydrate calories for energy.

Chemotherapy   Avoid eating your favorite foods within 24 hrs of
                  treatment to avoid negative associations with
                  them at a later time. Eat low-fat (less than 3 T or
                  40 g. fat/oil per day), high-carbohydrate (mainly
                  complex from grains, fruits, and vegetables) diet
                  with small quantities of good-quality protein.

AFTER TREATMENT:

Surgery   High-protein diet (8–10 oz. lean meat, poultry,
                  fish, or 2–3 eggs). Regular supplements as
                  above. Antioxidant supplement including 400
                  IU vitamin E and 1,000 mg. vitamin C per day.

Radiation	High-protein and -energy diet. Lactose-free and relatively low in simple sugars (sucrose, honey) to avoid intestinal discomfort.
Chemotherapy	Small, frequent meals of easy-to-digest foods such as fish, chicken, rice, baked potato, banana, applesauce. Stimulate appetite with ginger ale. If weight drops rapidly add energy drinks (see recipes) or meal replacement–type products. Avoid lactose as above.

SPECIFIC CHEMOTHERAPY AGENTS AND NUTRITION

Adriamycin	Interferes with riboflavin (vitamin B_2) activity. Be sure to include foods rich in B vitamins (wheat germ is a good source).
Adrucil (5FU)	Avoid fatty, spicy foods, alcohol, caffeine. Protein and glucose absorption is lowered, so eat small, frequent meals. Vitamin B_1 (thiamin) deficiency is possible (brown rice, wheat germ, lean meat are good sources of thiamin). There is some evidence that during 5FU treatment beta carotene is not recommended.
Bleomycin	Avoid megadose (more than 100% RDA) use of antioxidants, which may interfere with its action (antioxidants include beta carotene, vitamins C and E).
Cis or Carbo Platin	Avoid foods high in purines (organ meats, sardines, anchovies). Be sure to get sufficient magnesium (nuts, whole grains, dark green, leafy vegetables), potassium (bananas, mushrooms), and zinc (shellfish, whole grains), as needs increase also. *Drink plenty of water.*

Cytoxan

Avoid fatty foods. Eat small and frequent meals. Do not avoid sodium, as you may become sodium-deficient with this medication. *Drink plenty of water.*

Methotrexate

Avoid alcohol. Foods that produce an alkaline urine should be eaten to help excretion (almonds, buttermilk, chestnuts, coconuts, milk, fruits [except cranberries, prunes, and plums], vegetables [except corn and lentils]). Avoid excessive amounts of foods that produce acidic urine (nuts, meat, breads, and pasta). Since methotrexate is a folic acid antagonist, avoid megadose supplements (more than 100% RDA) of folic acid (a B vitamin). Leucovorin (folinic acid) is often given to enhance the effects of methotrexate.

Prednisone

Avoid excessive amounts of fatty foods and sodium-rich foods (processed foods, pickles, anchovies, canned soups and vegetables). Regular exercise will help normalize blood sugar levels, which may be more volatile with this medication. Fish oils provide vitamin D, which will help offset calcium depletion, another possible side effect of corticosteroids. Tuna, salmon, egg yolk, and fortified milk are also good sources of vitamin D (as is sunlight). Prevent potassium deficiencies by eating plenty of vegetables. Avoid laxatives, which can further deplete potassium. Always take prednisone with food to avoid gastrointestinal upset. Zinc, Vitamin B_6 and Vitamin C may also be compromised with this medication, so be sure to have a 100% RDA supplement of these daily.

Tamoxifen (Nolvadex)	Avoid excessive amounts of fatty foods and sodium-rich foods (processed foods, anchovies, canned soups and vegetables). Eat plenty of calcium- and magnesium-rich foods (fresh vegetables and nuts). Keep to a low-fat diet (less than 30% calories from fat) to avoid weight gain, an occasional side effect of tamoxifen.
Taxol	No special diet.
Vincristine (oncovin)	Avoid alcohol and caffeine. Drink plenty of fluids. Eat small quantities of easily digested foods. Do not avoid sodium, because even though you may have water retention, there may also be a sodium deficiency. Take a vitamin and mineral supplement because of possible malabsorption of nutrients. To avoid constipation eat plenty of insoluble fiber (wheat bran, brown rice, psyllium seed husks, Metamucil, etc.)

If your oncologist is using combinations of the above medications, modify the advice so that you retain the most important parts, e.g.,

CMF	Avoid fatty foods. Eat small quantities of bland flavors. Avoid alcohol, highly spiced foods, or very acidic foods (cranberries, pineapple, lemons, etc.). Focus on vegetables, on lean meats moistened in liquids, e.g., as stews or in soups, and on whole-grain cereals.

Many chemotherapy regimens affect your blood cell count. If not contraindicated, a hematinic (blood-building) supplement may be recommended. Check with your oncologist.

RADIATION TREATMENT AND NUTRITION

Radiation may affect your taste buds so that food may taste bitter or you may have a metallic taste in your mouth. Try marinating meats for better flavor. Cold foods may be more palatable than hot. Use herbs such as thyme, tarragon, mint, basil for added flavor. Try adding sauces such as applesauce, yogurt dressings, and salad dressings to make food easier to chew. Snack on protein-powder milk shakes (especially those made with soy protein, which contain anticarcinogens genistein and Bowman Burke Inhibitor). Ensure or other canned elemental diets are also useful standbys—look for low-sugar, high-fiber versions. For maximum effects, radiation treatment should not be combined with high-dose supplements of antioxidants (beta carotene, vitamins C and E, or glutathione). The amounts found in a normal mixed diet will not interfere with treatment. To counteract gastrointestinal problems, take additional B-complex vitamins as 9 tablets of brewer's yeast per day, or in a supplement. Four fl. oz. of aloe vera juice can also be a soothing drink. Avoid milk and milk products, as lactose intolerance may develop. Yogurt that uses a live culture may be tolerated well. You can use Lactaid milk and the Lactaid drops to minimize discomfort with dairy products. Ensure and similar meal-replacement drinks are lactose-free.

OTHER NUTRITIONAL IDEAS

Beta Carotene. This is a natural antioxidant which is nontoxic (although your skin may turn yellow if you take too much). Low serum levels have been shown to be associated with a higher mortality risk from lung cancer and there is other epidemiological evidence that this is a valuable protector from cell damage. It is found in cantaloupe melons, carrots, and dark green, leafy vegetables. Supplements derived from oceanic algae are sometimes recommended for cancer patients. There is some evidence that during chemotherapy for 5FU, supplemental beta carotene is not recommended.

Garlic. Allicin (allythio sulfinic allyl ester) is a weak anticancer agent found in garlic. Recognized as early as 1550 B.C. as a treatment for cancer.

Pycnogenol. This powerful antioxidant is found in grape seeds and in an extract from pine trees. Anyone with alcohol-related liver damage should not take this or megadoses of beta carotene for the same reasons.

Vitamins A and C. Foods rich in these vitamins provide antioxidant and anticarcinogenic activity. Examples are cantaloupe, mangoes, kiwi fruits, oranges, and carrots.

SOME IMPORTANT REMINDERS DURING TREATMENT

1. *Eat small amounts of food frequently (every couple of hours), rather than big meals. You may find your appetite is best in the morning, so have one good breakfast or two smaller ones.*

2. *Drink as much as you can (about 10–12 fl. cups), especially water, clear soups, and juices.*

3. *Imagine your digestion is like that of a young child. You can't eat a large quantity at one time and you can't digest some things. Small jars of weaning baby food may be helpful as ready-to-eat supplemental snack meals.*

4. *Microwaving or moist-cooking fruits and vegetables makes them more digestible. If fruits upset your stomach, use juices instead.*

5. *Experiment with different foods in small amounts—everyone's digestion is unique.*

NUTRITION AND IMMUNITY

Foods rich in the following nutrients are supportive to our immune system:

- Protein (lean meat, poultry, fish, eggs, milk, soy, and beans)
- Energy (complex carbohydrates, e.g., beans, whole grains)
- Essential fatty acids (fish, canola and olive oils, sunflower seeds)
- Vitamin A (liver, egg yolk) and Provitamin A beta carotene (carrots, cantaloupe, spinach)
- Vitamin B complex (wheat germ, liver, brewer's yeast)
- Vitamin C (citrus fruits, berries)
- Vitamin E (wheat germ, whole grains)
- Iron (red meat, liver, dark green, leafy vegetables, beans)
- Zinc (oysters, liver, sunflower seeds)
- Antioxidants (fruits, vegetables, whole grains)
- Anticarcinogens (cruciferous vegetables—broccoli, brussels sprouts, cabbage, cauliflower, kale, watercress)
- Garlic

PROTECTIVE FOODS:	DEFICIT FOODS:
dried apricots	sugar
bananas	alcohol
spinach	"empty calorie" foods, e.g., high-
carrots	fat, low-fiber foods like doughnuts
tomatoes	
strawberries	
blueberries	
blackberries	
raspberries	
onions	
brussels sprouts	
cabbage	
broccoli	

NATURAL ENERGY DRINKS

Many treatments for cancer can leave you feeling "low-energy." Food may taste bland and uninteresting. Here are some recipes to stimulate your appetite and give energy in a natural way.

ᘒ FRUIT SHAKE

> 1 cup plain low-fat yogurt
> 1 ripe banana
> a few drops vanilla extract
> 1 teaspoon honey
> 1 teaspoon coconut (optional)

Combine ingredients in a blender. The banana may be replaced with frozen strawberries, raspberries, half a papaya or mango, or a few chunks of pineapple.

ᘒ FRUIT JUICE SMOOTHY

> 2 cups apple juice
> 1 ripe banana
> ½ cup fresh or frozen berries
> ½ cup pineapple juice

Combine ingredients in a blender. Add ice if wished. Sip slowly with a straw.

ᘒ ENERGY DRINK: DRY MIX

> 1 cup peeled almonds
> 1 cup sesame seeds
> 2 tablespoons protein powder

Combine ingredients in a blender and blend until fine. This mix can be refrigerated for up to two weeks in a sealed jar.

∿ ENERGY DRINK: FRESH MIX

1 ripe banana
1 cup fruit juice (apple, cranberry, or similar)
½ cup mineral water
honey to taste (optional)

Combine ingredients with dry mix in blender. Sip slowly.
Remember—you can add fresh berries to give canned products (En-
sure, etc.) additional life.

IMMUNO-BROTH RECIPE

This is a vegetable-based soup that is high in immune-building
nutrients. It is easily digested and makes a filling meal despite being
low in calories. It is high in dietary fiber, which is supportive of
colon health. A diet consisting of 25–30 g. of fiber each day
improves the internal regulation of hormones. More than 35 g.
may interfere with mineral metabolism and is not recommended.

1 head of celery
1 bunch parsley
½ lb. green beans
4 zucchini
1 lb. fresh spinach, beet
    greens, or chard
½ green bell pepper
1 bunch scallions
1 large potato

3 carrots
½ head cauliflower or 1
    head broccoli
1 turnip/rutabaga
1 parsnip
2 cloves minced garlic
herbs to taste (thyme,
    oregano, marjoram,
    etc.)

Any other vegetables are possible—experiment with seasonal and
favorite varieties. Wash, slice, chop, or grate all the vegetables into
even-sized pieces. Place root vegetables (carrots, potatoes, turnip,
rutabaga, or parsnip) into a large pot. Half fill with water and bring
to a boil. Cover and simmer for 10 minutes. Add all the other

ingredients and season to taste. Return to a boil and cook for a further 1–2 minutes uncovered. Cover and simmer for a further 40 minutes. Adjust seasoning and serve hot or cold. This broth improves with age. Cool rapidly and keep refrigerated or freeze serving-sized portions for a quick meal. Make sure you reheat thoroughly and boil for at least 2 minutes when reheating. Tamari, soy sauce, or Bragg's liquid aminos improve the flavoring. You can add more carbohydrate energy by adding brown rice, barley, noodles, canned beans, or corn. Serve with hot bread. Makes 3–4 bowls.

There are many anticarcinogenic factors in vegetables which help your immune system. This soup is a good way of getting your daily protection. It contains less than 1 g. of fat.

SUGGESTIONS FOR HANDLING PROBLEMS DURING TREATMENT

Eat well to give you that extra edge as you participate in your own recovery. Choosing healthy foods is empowering, as you know you are doing your part by giving your body the nutrition that it needs to fight the cancer. Improved nutrition can also help you withstand the side effects of chemotherapy, radiation, and surgery. Some treatments may make eating difficult or distasteful. Here are some specific suggestions to help you with some of the most common treatment-related problems. Even if some of these suggestions are in conflict with the basic high-fiber/low–saturated fat concepts you are familiar with, maintaining a reasonably constant body weight is your overriding priority at this time.

Suggestions for chewing and swallowing difficulties:

1. Eat foods prepared with moist heat, e.g., soups, stews, eggs, pastas, quiches, casseroles.
2. Add gravy, sauces, butter, mayonnaise, or salad dressings to make food easier to swallow.

3. Avoid highly seasoned, spicy, tan or acidic foods (no citrus fruits, tomatoes, chilis).
4. Avoid alcohol and smoking.
5. Cold foods may be soothing if there are sores in the mouth.
6. Keep your caloric intake high by using meal replacement—type drinks, e.g., Ensure.
7. If you have trouble swallowing soups, try using a cup or glass instead of a spoon.

Suggestions for dealing with diarrhea:

1. Avoid high-fiber foods that contain a great deal of roughage, e.g., whole-wheat breads or cereals, raw fruits and vegetables except bananas, cooked vegetables with seeds or skins, dried beans and nuts, popcorn. Cucumber and lettuce may be difficult to digest also.
2. Eat water-soluble, fiber-rich foods, e.g., applesauce or puree, psyllium, e.g., Metamucil.
3. Don't drink *with* your meals, but plenty in between.
4. Eat frequent, small snack-type meals, rather than 3 large ones.
5. Food and liquids should be warm or at room temperature rather than very hot or ice cold.
6. For severe diarrhea restrict the diet to clear, warm liquids such as broth, flat ginger ale, or apple juice for one day. Check with your doctor if diarrhea persists more than one day.

Suggestions for dealing with nausea and/or vomiting:

1. Eat and drink slowly.
2. Eat small, frequent meals.
3. Avoid greasy, fatty, and fried foods.
4. Rest after meals.
5. For early morning or premeal nausea, try a cracker or dry toast.

6. Make up for lost calories when you feel more comfortable.
7. If cooking odors make you feel nauseated, try microwaving. Make sure a venting fan is on while you are cooking and eliminate especially unpleasant-smelling foods from your diet. Try frozen or chilled foods, as they give off less odor than warm ones.

Suggestions for loss of appetite:

1. If you aren't hungry at dinnertime, make breakfast or lunch your main meal. Similarly, if you aren't hungry first thing in the morning, eat more later in the day.
2. Eat more frequently, but smaller amounts of food.
3. Keep snacks readily available, e.g., in your purse or in the car.
4. Always make food look attractive with garnishes or with place settings.
5. Experiment with tastes—you may find things you didn't like before you like now.
6. Cold or room-temperature foods may be more appealing.
7. A glass of wine or beer may increase your appetite (check with your doctor first in case alcohol doesn't mix with a medication).
8. Increase the caloric intake of the foods you do eat with a small amount of "light" (less strongly flavored, not lower in calories) olive oil.
9. Try some of the commercially prepared food supplements, e.g., Ensure, Sustacal, or Polycose, available from most good pharmacies or drugstores. Add fresh berries or juice for variety and additional botanical factors.

SUGGESTIONS FOR EATING FOR MAXIMUM IMMUNITY

By making wise eating choices you may be able to fortify your natural defenses and handle treatments with ease. Remember also to take extra care with personal and foot hygiene at this time. Listen to your body's needs for rest and sleep. You will benefit from being in natural surroundings and keeping company with those who don't drain you of energy.

As each person's nutritional needs are very individual, I suggest that you see a nutritionist or dietitian at this time to assist you in making healthy food choices. The following foods are sources of nutrients that your body needs to maintain its immunity.

NUTRIENT FOR IMMUNITY:	FOOD SOURCE:
Vitamin A	Fish liver oils, liver
Beta carotene (Pro vitamin A)	Orange, yellow, and dark green, leafy vegetables including carrots, cantaloupe, apricots, broccoli, spinach
Vitamin B_2 (Riboflavin)	Whole and enriched cereals and breads; lean meat, milk, eggs, liver, dried yeast
Vitamin B_6 (Pyridoxine)	As for B_2, plus bananas
Folic acid	Leafy, green vegetables, meats
Pantothenic acid	Brewer's yeast, legumes, salmon, whole grains
Vitamin C	Citrus fruits, berries, broccoli, bell peppers
Vitamin E	Leafy, green vegetables, egg yolk, liver, wheat germ
Selenium	Garlic, legumes, fish, asparagus

Iron	Liver, peas, egg yolk, asparagus
Magnesium	Green, leafy vegetables, nuts, seafood
Manganese	Bananas, bran, celery, pineapple, nuts
Protein	Lean meat, poultry, fish, shellfish, eggs, legumes, broccoli, sunflower seeds
Antioxidants	Citrus fruits, legumes, whole grains

DIETARY FAT AND CANCER

Recent studies are indicating that hormone-related cancers (breast, colorectal, and prostate) are linked to a high dietary animal-fat and protein intake. It is prudent to cut back to 15% of your calories from fat with only 5% coming from animal sources (butter, milk, yogurt, meat, etc.) and 10% from vegetables (oils, avocados, olives). Remember that too little fat is also harmful and if you go lower than 15% of your calories from fat (about 1–2 T oil per day), then use a supplement of borage or flaxseed oil for essential fatty acids.

If you have been diagnosed with another type of cancer it is prudent to eat about 20–25% of your calories from fat with a similar ratio of less than ⅓ from animal sources.

FAT CONTENT OF VARIOUS FOODS

HIGH   (50–100% OF CALORIES DERIVED FROM FAT)

100%   Butter, margarine, vegetable oils, mayonnaise

95%   Whipping cream, olives, pecans

90%   Cream cheese, Italian dressing, avocado

85%   Hot dog, pork sausage, sour cream, Thousand Island
           dressing, walnuts

80%   Bacon, spareribs, half-and-half

75%   Cashews, cheddar cheese, lamb chops, peanut butter,
           salami, sunflower seeds, T-bone steak (untrimmed)

70%   Ham, pork chops (including edge), Swiss cheese, Vel-
           veeta

65%   Eggs (whole), ice cream, potato salad

60%   Chocolate (sweet German)

55%   Granola, T-bone steak (trimmed)

MEDIUM   **(30–50% OF CALORIES FROM FAT)**

45%   Milk (3.5%), doughnuts, custard, french fries, oil-
           packed tuna, "granola" cereals, tofu, chocolate chip
           cookies

40%   Creamed cottage cheese, skinless poultry, commercial
           taco shells, pork chops (trimmed), salmon

35%   Low-fat (2%) milk, Swiss and American cheese slices,
           flank steak, lamb (trimmed), cheese pizza (thin crust)

30%   Beef bouillon, ice milk, corn bread, low-fat muffins

LOW   **(BELOW 30% OF CALORIES FROM FAT)**

25%   Raw oysters, saltine crackers, low-fat chocolate milk,
           medium-fat yogurt (2–5 g. fat per serving), low-fat
           (1%) milk

20%   Graham crackers and most low-fat crackers, low-fat
           (2%) cottage cheese, low-fat yogurt

15%   Corn and flour tortillas, most bread, water-packed tuna, fresh white fish

<10%   Fruits and vegetables, cereals, low-fat yogurt, low-calorie salad dressings, skim (nonfat) milk, shrimp, crab, lobster, chocolate syrup

NO FAT

Sherbet, rice, most pastas, hard candy, egg white, most fruits and vegetables

APPENDIX 4

Script for Directed Visualization

This script should be read slowly and deliberately into a tape recorder in your normal voice. Pause periodically so that when you listen to the tape, you will have time to absorb the instructions.

PROCEDURE FOR LISTENING TO THE TAPE

- Allot about twenty minutes twice a day.
- Sit or lie quietly where you can be alone and quiet for that period of time. Play the tape. It contains all the directions.
- Make a conscious effort to follow the directions.

SCRIPT FOR DIRECTED VISUALIZATION

This is going to be a time of complete relaxation . . . a conscious effort to relax as completely as possible. Get into as comfortable a position as you can, and close your eyes. For the next couple of minutes, just concentrate on your breathing. To the best of your ability, see your lungs . . . see how they feel, consciously see how they feel while they're completely expanded, and see how they feel after you exhale. Be aware that there's no right way and no wrong way to do what you're doing now . . . that whatever results you get are perfect results, and that if all you do is relax, that's wonderful. This is not a time to be worrying about any of the things that are happening in your day-to-day life. This is a time only for you, and you can let it all hang out. For this very short period of time, you can completely relax. You are never out of control. You can feel completely secure.

Now, once again, concentrate on your lungs. Picture them in your mind's eye. See if you can see them filled . . . see if you can see them after you relax. And if your mind drifts away, and you want to, just bring it slowly back to where you are or where you want it to be. You are doing nothing wrong, and anything you do will be a success. And if you hear my voice, that'll be fine . . . and if you don't, that's fine too. You can be absolutely sure that your subconscious is hearing every word I say.

And now perhaps, in your mind's eye—way, way out in space—you can see a word all lit up . . . and the word is *relax*. Just relax . . . and now that same word is about a foot in front of your forehead . . . just see it about a foot in front of your forehead, the word *relax*. And now inside your forehead, see that word, and just relax.

Now perhaps, if you want to, pay attention to your left foot, and the toes on your left foot, and your ankle, and let them all relax . . . and all the cares and tensions of the day just drain down into the floor. Consciously let them relax . . . and any noise you hear will only serve to deepen your relaxation.

And now pay attention, if you will, to your right shoulder. All the muscles of your right shoulder, completely relaxed. All the cares of the day drain away and leave you. And consciously check your right shoulder to see if there's any tension there. Think about it. And now all the muscles and tendons of your right foot, and the toes of your right foot, and the ankle, just let them relax. And now the calf of your right leg, let it relax. And for this very short time in your mind's eye, perhaps you can see that wonderfully long bone running from your ankle to your knee in your right leg . . . see how wonderfully straight and long and solid it is . . . and what a wonderful feat of construction. Let it relax . . . let all the muscles just relax . . . and the muscles of your left calf . . . relax. And way, way out in the future, and way, way into the past.

And this is a process just like when you were a very, very little person and you didn't know how to ride a bicycle, or tell time, or read. And when you were out learning to ride a bicycle, you couldn't even tell how long you were out there because you couldn't tell time, and you didn't know whether there was a difference between writing and printing . . . and this is also a learning process . . . learning to relax . . . learning to be at ease.

And now let all the muscles of your left shoulder completely relax . . . let it just droop toward the ground . . . and rest comfortably against the seat you're in. Let it relax. And now the muscles of your stomach. Let your stomach just hang out . . . just relaxed. Once again, it's like when you were a very, very little person, just learning how to do all the things you had to do, like telling time and reading . . . And now the muscles of your left thigh . . . This is a time for relaxation . . . and you don't have to go to sleep . . . but if you do, that's fine . . . and if my voice drifts away, that's fine . . . and if your mind drifts away, that's fine too. Whatever you do is wonderful. Completely relax.

And now all the muscles of the right thigh . . . just let them relax. All the tensions of the day just drain out of them into the seat below you. And there's that word *relax*. Consciously in your mind is the word *relax,* way, way out in the past . . . just in the past . . . and right behind your forehead.

And all the muscles of your face now . . . the muscles of your lips, your cheeks, and your forehead . . . just let them fall toward the ground and your stomach. And your chest . . . once again, your chest just relaxed, and now your back, and your complete right arm and the fingers of your right hand. And if there's any part of your body that's not completely relaxed already, it soon will be.

You may be surprised to see how relaxed you are already. That may come as a surprise to you . . . and as I said, if there's any part of your body that's not yet relaxed, it soon will be. And if there's any part of your body that's not feeling as comfortable as it might, concentrate on that part of the body for the next few seconds . . .

just think of it . . . and send all the endorphins★ of the brain down in that area. Consciously be aware of any part of your body that's not as comfortable as it might be.

And now all the muscles and sinews and tendons of your left arm and your left hand and the fingers of your left hand completely relax. And all the muscles of your neck and your shoulders and your chest and your buttocks and the whole pelvic area now . . . Think about the whole pelvic area . . . once again your face . . . and your head . . . And if my voice drifts away, that's fine, just as long as you're sitting back comfortably and relaxing. Many things are changing in your body, all of which are normal and wonderful, just through your relaxation.

And now perhaps, if you want to, you'll see yourself at the top of a flight of ten steps going down. You've been at the top of stairs before, and you will be again. So this is completely familiar to you. This is a time when you can just put your trust in the world. You will never be out of control in any way. You can trust . . . like you did when you were a very, very little person. And everything is going to turn out exactly as you want it to. We're going to walk down these steps together, if you want to, and with every step down you take, you're going to relax just a little bit more.

And now, if you will, you can take the first step down . . . and you've taken one step down, and you have nine to go. And with every step down, you relax just a little bit more. And any noise you hear will serve to relax you just a little bit more. And way, way out in the future, and way, way back in the past, and right behind your forehead is that word *relax*.

And now, you take another step down. And with every step down, you relax just a little bit more, and now you have taken two steps down, and you have eight steps to go and take another step down . . . relaxing just a little bit more with every step you go down. And feel that relaxation in your body . . . You may be surprised at how relaxed you feel already. And now take another

★ Endorphins are painkilling chemicals that occur naturally in the brain.

step down, and that's four steps down, and you have six to go. This is a time for relaxation. It's not necessary for you to go to sleep, but if you want to, that's fine. If it happens, that's fine; or if your mind drifts away, that's fine. Nothing that you do is wrong.

Take one more step down. And now you're halfway down the stairs . . . You have five more steps to go . . . and you take another step down. And see yourself, consciously see yourself on the sixth step down, and how comfortable you feel, and how secure you feel, and how trusting you feel. And now another step down . . . and now you've taken seven steps down and you have three to go. And there's that word *relax* shining way, way out in the heavens and behind your forehead at the same time . . . and you take another step down . . . and you've taken eight steps and you have two more to go. And now one more step . . . and you've taken nine steps down and you have one to go . . . and now take that last step down, and you're all the way down to the bottom of the stairs. And you may be surprised at how relaxed you really are.

And now, if you want to, and it's easy for you to do . . . perhaps you can see yourself on a lovely, lovely, warm, comfortable beach. And way out in front of you is a calm, calm, very blue ocean. Very calm and very blue. And see if you can smell what the ocean smells like. Really try to smell it. Be there. And the sun is just beating down on your body in a way that can't hurt you under any circumstances . . . and feel the cool breeze over your body and how comfortable that feels. And hear the ocean lapping on the shore. Listen to what it sounds like. And underneath your feet is the warm sand, just the right temperature, the way you like it best. And behind you is an enormous beach, friendly and protective and just wonderful.

And now, while you're standing there, perhaps you can see yourself as a very, very little person at a time when you were very happy, very content, and very secure. And feel that happiness, and feel that security, and feel that carefree feeling, and know that that's you . . . And remember that any noise you hear will just relax you further. And you can call back this feeling of happiness and contentment anytime you want to . . . it's *your* feeling and it's *your* memory. The only one in the world who has that memory is you.

And now, if you want to, see yourself standing on the beach once again, as an adult . . . And now, if you want to, knowing that there's a large, comfortable beach towel on the beach to guard your head, see yourself lie down on your back and feel how secure the ground is under you, holding your calves and your backside and your shoulders and your head. Feel how secure that is.

And now, perhaps you'll see yourself surrounded by a lovely golden light. It covers every inch of your body while all the normal functions go on . . . You breathe very normally and your pores are open, and every normal function goes on. And that lovely, lovely golden light is a combination of all the healing power of the universe, and all the healing power of your own body, and all the healing power of any medication you're taking or radiation you're receiving, or anything you're taking . . . and that golden light can go anyplace you tell it to.

And now, if you want to, see that part of your body that is not exactly as you want it to be. And direct that golden light to go to that part of your body and surround that area or areas. And know that the golden light surrounding the part of your body that is not as healthy as you want it to be combines all the healing power of the universe, and all the healing power in your body, and all the healing power of any medication that you're taking. It's an extraordinarily powerful elixir. And any cancer cells that are there are weak and erratic cells and easily defeated. And you can tell the golden light to crush any cancer cells, and to diminish any tumor . . . and to do anything you want it to do . . . and it's a powerful, vital, vigorous force and the cancer cells are weak and erratic.

Consciously see the golden light surrounding all of the area where your body is not in the condition you want it to be. And notice . . . notice how it can bring the endorphins of your brain down into that area and soothe any pain . . . and help to alleviate any problem that's going on in your body. And tell that golden light to do what you want it to do. It is *your* golden light. It is going to go where you want it to. And by telling it where you want it to go, you can take some charge of your body.

And now, I'm going to be quiet for a minute or two, and while I'm quiet, perhaps you'll want to continue to think about that golden light doing all the things you want it to do. I'm going to be quiet starting now. [*Pause for sixty seconds.*]

And now, with that golden light still within you . . . that powerful, vigorous, vital golden light still within you, that golden light that combines all the power of the universe and of your body, and of any medication or radiation or anything else you're taking . . . with all of that still within you . . . and completely at your command . . . from now and forever . . . perhaps you'll see yourself stand up on the beach. And as you stand on the beach, if you want to . . . visualize yourself without any physical problem whatsoever, and see what feeling comes over you without any physical problem whatsoever. And know that that's *your* feeling and that you can call on that feeling at any time. You can call on that feeling, or you can call on the golden light, or you can call on the feeling of security at any time without interfering in any way with all of the things that you're doing.

And now perhaps, if you'd like, see yourself at the bottom of the same flight of stairs you just came down, and we'll walk up those stairs together. When you reach the top of the stairs, you will be back at a place where you started, feeling completely alert, at least as well as you felt when we started, and most likely much better . . . and take the first step up. And now the second step up [*speak slowly here*] . . . and the third, and the fourth, and the fifth . . . and you're halfway up . . . and when you reach the tenth step, you'll be back in the place where you started, feeling completely alert and at least as well as you felt when you started and, perhaps and most likely, much better.

And now you can open your eyes at any time. And now, take the next step up, and you're back at the place where you started . . . feeling completely alert and at least as well as you felt when you started, and most likely much better . . . and you can open your eyes at any time.

APPENDIX 5

◯◡

The Wellness Community Facilities

National: 2716 Ocean Park Blvd., Suite 1040, Santa Monica, CA 90405
  • President—Harold H. Benjamin, Ph.D. • Vice President, Program Director—Mitch Golant, Ph.D. • Chairperson—David E. Gooding • 310-314-2555 • Fax 310-314-7586

Ben and Joyce Eisenberg National Training Center: 2716 Ocean Park Blvd., Suite 1040, Santa Monica, CA 90405
  • Program Director—Michael States, M.A., MFCC
  • Opened June 1982 • Visits per month—737 • 310-314-2555 • Fax 310-314-7586

Baltimore: Dulaney Center II, 901 Dulaney Valley Road, #710, Baltimore, MD 21204
  • Executive Director—Suzanne K. Brace, M.S. • Program Director—Tom Large, LCSW • Chairperson—Erwin Huber • Opened April 1993 • Visits per month—225
  • 410-832-2719 • Fax 410-337-0937

Greater Boston: 1320 Centre Street, #305, Newton Centre, MA 02159
  • Executive Director—Mary Ellen Stowell • Program Director—Pamela Narrett-Willsey, LISCW • Chairperson—Marcy Balter • Opened September 1993 • Visits per month—408
  • 617-332-1919 • Fax 617-332-2727

Greater Cincinnati: Towers of Kenwood, 8044 Montgomery Road, #385, Cincinnati, OH 45236

• Executive Director—Lynn Stern • Program Director—Don Smith, LISW • Chairperson—Terry Bruck • Opened November 1990 • Visits per month—711
• 513-791-4060 • Fax 513-791-8239

Foothills: 200 E. Del Mar, Suite 118, Pasadena, CA 91105
• Executive Director—Anne Kennedy, M.S., M.B.A. • Program Director—Carolyn M. Loper, MFCC • Chairperson—Joseph R. Henry • Opened August 1990 • Visits per month—533
• 818-796-1083 • Fax 818-796-4685

Knoxville: 1844 Terrace Avenue, Knoxville, TN 37916
• Administrative Director—Sandra McCarrell, M.S. • Program Director—LeAnne Dougherty, LCSW, D.S.W. • Chairperson—David White • Opened January 1990 • Visits per month–190
• 615-546-4661 • Fax 615-522-1912

Orange County: 1924 E. Glenwood Place, Santa Ana, CA 92705
• Executive Director—Shirley Lorenz • Program Director—Barbara McKone, Ph.D. • Chairperson—Hugh Saddington • Opened August 1990 • Visits per month—414
• 714-258-1210 • Fax 714-258-0806

Philadelphia: 4610 City Line Avenue, Philadelphia, PA 19131
• Executive Director—Constance M. Carino, R.N., DNSc • Program Director—Lori Mossberg Curtis, M.S.W. • Chairperson—Jack Wilkie • Opened June 1993 • Visits per month—275
• 215-879-7733 • Fax 215-879-6575

Greater St. Louis: 10425 Old Olive Street Road, Suite 202, St. Louis, MO 63141
• Executive Director—Barbara J. Henning, M.S.W., LCSW • Program Director—Greg Pacini, M.S., L.P.C. • Chairperson—Mel Dunkelman • Opened September 1993 • Visits per month—243
• 314-993-4333 • Fax 314-993-6835

San Diego: 8555 Aero Drive, #340, San Diego, CA 92123
• Executive Director—Jan Allen • Program Director—Margaret

Stauffer, MFCC • Chairperson—Richard Bigelow • Opened January 1990 • Visits per month—554
• 619-467-1065 • Fax 619-467-1082

S.F. East Bay: 350 No. Wiget Lane, #101, Walnut Creek, CA 94598
• Executive Director—Charles B. McNeil • Program Director—Shannon McGowan, MFCC • Chairperson—Stephen D. Roath • Opened September 1990 • Visits per month—715
• 510-933-0107 • Fax 510-933-0249

South Bay Cities: 109 W. Torrance Blvd., #100, Redondo Beach, CA 90277
• Executive Director—Judith K. Howe • Program Director—Marya Foley, M.A., MFCC • Chairperson—Michael Moorhead • Opened April 1987 • Visits per month—598
• 310-376-3550 • Fax 310-372-2094

Valley/Ventura: 530 Hampshire Road, Thousand Oaks, CA 91361
• Executive Director—Suzanne Wedow, Ph.D. • Program Director—Marty Nason, R.N., M.N. • Chairperson—Leonard M. Linton • Opened June 1991 • Visits per month—311
• 805-379-4777 • Fax 805-371-6231

Inland Valley: 8976 Foothill Blvd., B-7, Suite 225, Rancho Cucamonga, CA 91730
• Chairperson—Phyllis La Plante
• 909-715-2530

Delaware: P.O. Box 4665, Wilmington, DE 19807
• Director—Ellen Hamilton • Chairperson—Cynthia C. Dwyer
• 302-656-8410

West Florida: 1345 Main Street, Suite C4, Sarasota, FL 34236
• Chairperson—Cheri Krumholz
• 813-957-3561 • Fax 813-955-7364

Atlanta: 3261 Lenox Road, Atlanta, GA 30324
• Director—Marcia Greenburg • Chairperson—Sandy Zatcoff
• 404-814-0050 • Fax 404-814-0043

Central Indiana: 8465 Keystone Crossing, #242, Indianapolis, IN 46240
  • Director—Vicki Kennedy • Chairperson—Edgar Goldwasser
  • 317-257-1505

Northwest Ohio: 842 W. South Boundary, Perrysburg, OH 43551
  • Director—Sue Muller • Chairperson—Jacquie Boynton
  • 419-872-0377 • Fax 419-872-2070

APPENDIX 6

Additional Resources

American Brain Tumor Association
2720 River Road, Suite 146
Des Plaines, IL 60018
800-886-2282

Offers free services including publications about brain tumors, support group lists, referral information, and a pen pal program.

American Cancer Society (ACS)
1599 Clifton Road, N.E.
Atlanta, GA 30329
800-ACS-2345
Reach to Recovery I Can Cope
Road to Recovery
International Association of Laryngectomees
Look Good, Feel Better
Resources, Information and Guidance (RIG)

Dedicated to eliminating cancer as a major health problem through research, education, and service.

American Foundation for Urologic Disease
300 West Pratt Street, Suite 401
Baltimore, MD 21201-2463
800-242-2383
Bladder Health Council
Prostate Health Council
Prostate Cancer Survivors Network

Provides educational information for the public, patients, and health care professionals about urologic diseases.

American Institute for Cancer Research (AICR)
1759 R Street NW
Washington, D.C. 20069
800-843-8114 (Nutrition Hotline)
202-328-7744 (in Washington, D.C.)

The AICR is the only major national cancer organization that supports research and provides public education exclusively in the area of diet nutrition and cancer. Offers free publications.

American Lung Association
1740 Broadway
New York, NY 10019-4374
212-315-8700 • Fax
212-265-5642

Dedicated to conquering lung disease and promoting lung health.

Biological Therapy Institute Foundation
P.O. Box 681700
Franklin, TN 37068
615-790-7535 • Fax
615-794-9110

A leading resource for physician and patient information regarding the use of biopharmaceuticals in cancer therapy.

R. A. Bloch Cancer Foundation, Inc.
The Cancer Hotline
4410 Main Street
Kansas City, MO 64111
816-932-8453

Helps people diagnosed with cancer have the best possibility of beating it as easily as possible through informational resources, peer counseling, medical second opinions, and support groups.

Bone Marrow Transplant (BMT) Newsletter
1985 Spruce Avenue
Highland Park, IL 60035
708-831-1913

Publishes bimonthly newsletter and a book on issues of concern to patients. Provides attorney referrals for those having difficulty obtaining reimbursement for their treatment.

Bone Marrow Transplant Family Support Network
P.O. Box 845
Avon, CT 06001
800-826-9376

Enables families to feel "connected" when coping with the decision, daily routines prior to and following transplants, and follow-up care after a transplant.

Burger King Cancer Caring Center
4117 Liberty Avenue
Pittsburgh, PA 15224
412-622-1212

Dedicated to helping people diagnosed with cancer, their families and friends cope with the emotional impact of cancer. The Cancer Caring Center is now handling calls for the Cancer Guidance Hotline.

Cancer Care, Inc.
1180 Avenue of the Americas
New York, NY 10036
212-221-3300

Offers professional social work, counseling, and guidance to help patients and families cope with the emotional and psychological consequences of cancer.

Cancer Conquerors Foundation
P.O. Box 238
Hershey, PA 17033
800-238-6479 or 717-533-6124

Offers cancer survival training programs and self-study materials with specific emphasis on body/mind/spirit integration.

CAN ACT (Cancer Patients Action Alliance)
26 College Place
Brooklyn, NY 11201
718-522-4607

Provides advocacy and public policy, but does not provide services for individuals.

Cancer Research Institute
681 Fifth Avenue
New York, NY 10022
212-688-7515 or 800-99-CANCER
Fax 212-832-9376

Supports leading-edge research aimed at developing new methods of diagnosing, treating, and preventing cancer.

Cancer Support Network
Essex House, Suite L10
Baum Blvd. at South Negley Avenue
Pittsburgh, PA 15206-3703
412-361-8600

Provides emotional and psychological support through peer support groups, educational programs, community workshops, advocacy, and social gatherings.

Cancervive
6500 Wilshire Blvd., Suite 500
Los Angeles, CA 90048
310-203-9232

Assists cancer survivors to face and overcome the challenges of "Life After Cancer."

Candlelighters Childhood Cancer Foundation
7910 Woodmont Avenue, Suite 460
Bethesda, MD 20814-3015
800-366-2223 or 301-657-8401

Provides information, support, and advocacy to families of children with cancer, survivors of childhood cancer, and professionals who work with them.

ChemoCare
231 North Avenue West
Westfield, NJ 07090
800 55-CHEMO (outside NJ)
908-233-1103 (inside NJ)

Offers personal one-to-one emotional support to cancer patients and their families undergoing chemotherapy and/or radiation treatment, from trained and certified volunteers who have survived the treatment themselves.

The Chemotherapy Foundation
183 Madison Avenue, Suite 403
New York, NY 10016
212-213-9292

Supports laboratory and clinical research to develop more effective methods of diagnosis and therapy for the control and cure of cancer. Conducts professional and public education programs and provides free patient/public information booklets.

Children's Oncology Camps of America
c/o Linda Wells
7 Richland Memorial Park, Suite 203
Columbia, SC 29203
803-434-3533

Provides normal life experiences for children, their siblings, and their families.

Choice in Dying
200 Varick Street, Room 1001
New York, NY 10014-4810
800-989-WILL

Advocates the recognition and protection of individual rights at the end of life. Provides counseling for individuals regarding preparing and using advance directives and durable powers of attorney for health care.

Coping Magazine
2019 North Carothers
Franklin, TN 37064
615-790-2400 • Fax
615-791-4719

A bimonthly publication which is the only nationally distributed consumer magazine for people whose lives have been touched by cancer.

Corporate Angel Network (CAN)
Westchester County Airport
Building 1
White Plains, NY 10604
914-328-1313

Helps cancer patients bridge the miles between home and needed treatment using corporate aircraft.

Encore Plus
YWCA of the U.S.A.
624 9th Street NW, 3rd Floor
Washington, D.C. 20001-5394
202-628-3636

Postoperative program for women, consisting of peer support and exercise.

**Families Against Cancer
(FACT)**
P.O. Box 588
DeWitt, NY 13214
315-446-5326 • 315-446-6385

*Advocacy agency which provides
information to the public that justifies
increasing federal dollars to research
cancer for early diagnosis and
intervention and provides educational
materials on cancer prevention and
intervention.*

Friends Network
P.O. Box 4545
Santa Barbara, CA 93140
805-565-7031

*A national nonprofit organization
offering the only national cancer
activities newsletter in color*—The
Funletter, *which benefits children
with cancer.*

**International Myeloma
Foundation**
2120 Stanley Hills Drive
Los Angeles, CA 90046
800-452-CURE

*Promotes education for physicians and
patients about myeloma, its treatment
and management. Funds research,
holds clinical and scientific conferences,
publishes a quarterly newsletter,*
Myeloma Today.

**Susan G. Komen Breast
Cancer Foundation**
5005 LBJ Freeway, Suite 370
Dallas, TX 75244
800 IM AWARE (800-462-9273)

*Dedicated to eradicating breast cancer
as a life-threatening disease by
advancing research, education,
screening, and treatment.*

Leukemia Society of America
600 Third Avenue
New York, NY 10016
800-955-4LSA (educational
materials)
212-573-8484 (general
information)

*Dedicated to seeking the cause and
eventual cure of leukemia and related
cancers. Nationwide programs include
research, patient aid, public and professional education. Offers local fam-
ily-support-group programs free of
charge, open to patients, families,
and friends.*

**Lymphoma Research
Foundation of America, Inc.**
2318 Prosser Avenue
Los Angeles, CA 90064
310-470-4912

*A research organization that also
provides a support system for
lymphoma patients across the country.*

Make Today Count
c/o Connie Zimmerman
Mid America Cancer Center
1235 E. Cherokee
Springfield, MO 65804-2263
800-432-2273

*A mutual support organization that
brings together persons affected by a
life-threatening illness so they may
help each other.*

**The Mautner Project For
Lesbians With Cancer**
1707 L Street NW, Suite 1060
Washington, D.C. 20036
202-332-5536

*Provides vital services and support,
including education, information, and
advocacy for health issues relating to
lesbians with cancer and their families.*

**National Alliance of Breast
Cancer Organizations
(NABCO)**
9 East 37th Street, 10th Floor
New York, New York 10016
212-719-4154

*Source of information on breast cancer.
Advocates for legislative and regulatory
concerns of breast cancer community.*

**National Bone Marrow
Transplant Link (BMT Link)**
29209 Northwestern Hwy.,
#624
Southfield, MI 48034
800-LINK-BMT

*Reduces the burdens of those affected
by bone marrow transplantation and
promotes public understanding and
peer support.*

**National Brain Tumor
Foundation**
785 Market Street, Suite 16
San Francisco, CA 94103
800-934-CURE

*Pursues two major goals: providing
support and education for brain tumor
patients and finding a cure through
research.*

**National Breast Cancer
Coalition**
1707 L Street NW, Suite 1060
Washington, D.C. 21036
202-296-7477 • Fax
202-265-6854

*A grass-roots advocacy movement of
more than 300 member organizations
and thousands of individuals working
through a national action network,
dedicated to the eradication of breast
cancer through action, policy, and
advocacy.*

**National Cancer Institute
(NCI) Cancer Information
Service**
Building 31, Room 10A16
9000 Rockville Pike
Bethesda, MD 20892
800-4-CANCER
301-402-5874 CANCERFAX

Provides a nationwide telephone service for cancer patients and their families and friends, the public, and health care professionals that answers questions and sends booklets about cancer. CANCERFAX provides treatment guidelines, with current data on prognosis, relevant staging and histologic classifications, news and announcements of important cancer-related issues. Call CANCERFAX from your fax machine.

National Cancer Survivors Day (NCSD) Foundation

2819 North Carothers, Suite 100
Franklin, TN 37064
615-794-3006 • Fax
615-791-4719

NCSD is America's nationwide annual celebration of life, for cancer survivors, their families, friends, and oncology teams. NCSD is celebrated on the first Sunday in June of each year in communities throughout America.

National Coalition for Cancer Research (NCCR)

426 C Street NE
Washington, D.C. 20002
202-544-1880

Educates the public and elected officials about the need to provide a supportive environment for the successful implementation of the National Cancer Act.

National Coalition for Cancer Survivorship (NCCS)

1010 Wayne Avenue, 5th Floor
Silver Spring, MD 20910
301-650-8868

Dedicated to enhancing the quality of life for cancer survivors and promoting an understanding of cancer survivorship.

National Hospice Organization (NHO)

1901 N. Moore Street, Suite 901
Arlington, VA 22209
800-658-8898

A resource for hospice professionals, volunteers, and the general public for terminally ill patients and their families.

National Kidney Cancer Association

1234 Sherman Avenue, Suite 200
Evanston, IL 60202
708-332-1051

Works to increase the survival of kidney cancer patients and improve their care by providing information, sponsoring research, and acting as an advocate on behalf of patients.

National Lymphedema Network

221 I Post Street, Suite 404
San Francisco, CA 94115
800-541-3259

Disseminates information on the prevention and management of primary and secondary lymphedema to the general public as well as health care professionals.

National Marrow Donor Program
3433 Broadway Street NE, Suite 400
Minneapolis, MN 55413
800-MARROW-2

A congressionally authorized network which maintains a computerized data bank of available tissue-typed marrow-donor volunteers nationwide.

Oley Foundation
214 Hun Memorial
Albany Medical Center A-23
Albany, NY 12208
800-776-OLEY

Support for home parenteral and/or enteral nutrition therapy consumers and their families through a newsletter, conferences, meetings, outreach, and support activities.

PDQ (Physician Data Query)
800-4-CANCER

PDQ is the National Cancer Institute's computerized listing of up-to-date and accurate information for patients and health professionals on the latest types of cancer treatments, research studies, clinical trials, new

and promising cancer treatments, and organizations and doctors involved in caring for people with cancer. To access PDQ, doctors may use an office computer or the services of a medical library. Doctors and patients can also get information by calling the above number.

Patient Advocates for Advanced Cancer Treatments (PAACT)
1143 Parmelee NW
Grand Rapids, MI 49504
616-453-1477

An association for both patients and physicians for diagnostic and therapeutic treatments of prostate cancer.

Ronald McDonald Houses
One Kroc Drive
Oak Brook, IL 60521
708-575-7418

Offers a refuge from the hospital, a "home away from home."

The Skin Cancer Foundation
245 Fifth Avenue, Suite 2402
New York, NY 10016
212-725-5176

Provides public and medical education programs and support for medical training and research. Helps reduce incidence, morbidity, and mortality of skin cancer.

Support for People with Oral and Head and Neck Cancer, Inc. (SPOHNC)

P.O. Box 53
Locust Valley, NY 11560-0053
516-759-5333

*Self-help program of support.
Addresses the broad emotional,
psychological, and humanistic needs
of these cancer survivors, empowering
each to take an active role in his or
her recovery.*

United Ostomy Association, Inc.

36 Executive Park, Suite 120
Irvine, CA 92714
714-660-8624 or 800-826-0826

*Association of ostomy chapters
dedicated to complete rehabilitation of
all ostomates.*

US TOO International, Inc.

930 North York Road, Suite 50
Hinsdale, IL 60521-2993
708-323-1002 or 800-808-7866
Fax 708-323-1003

*Provides prostate cancer survivors and
their families emotional and
educational support through an
international network of chapters.*

The Wellness Community

2716 Ocean Park Blvd., Suite 1040
Santa Monica, CA 90405-5211
310-314-2555

*Provides free psychosocial support to
people fighting to recover from cancer
as an adjunct to conventional medical
treatment. Thirteen facilities
nationwide.*

Y-ME

National Breast Cancer
Organization
212 W. Van Buren, 4th Floor
Chicago, IL 60607
800-221-2141
312-986-8228 (24-hour hotline)

*Hotline counseling, educational
programs, and self-help meetings for
breast cancer patients, their families
and friends.*

Y-Me Men's Support Line
Monday–Friday, 9 A.M.–5 P.M.
CST

*Men can call the Y-Me 800 number
and request to speak to a male
counselor. The counselor most closely
matched in experience to the caller
will return the call within 24 hours.*

[Editor's Note: *The above listing
represents organizations that operate
on a national level. There are many
excellent local organizations too
numerous to list. To locate them, call
your local cancer treatment center, or
local American Cancer Society office.*]
Reprinted by permission of Coping
magazine.

BIBLIOGRAPHY

American Cancer Society. *Cancer Facts and Figures for 1994*. New York: American Cancer Society, 1994.

Bahnson, C. B. "Psychosomatic Issues in Cancer," in *The Psycho-somatic Approach to Illness*, R. L. Gallon, ed. New York: Elsevier Biomedical, 1982.

Benjamin, Harold H. *From Victim to Victor*. Los Angeles: J. P. Tarcher, 1989.

Benson, Herbert. "The Placebo Effect." *Harvard Medical School Health Letter*, August 1980, pp. 3–4.

Benson, Herbert. *The Relaxation Response*. New York: William Morrow, 1975.

Berkman, Lisa E. and Breslow, Lester. *Health and Ways of Living*. New York: Oxford University Press, 1983.

Borysenko, Joan. "Psychoneuroimmunology: Behavioral Factors and the Immune Response." *ReVision*, 7 (Spring 1984), pp. 56–65.

Brown, Barbara. *New Mind, New Body*. New York: Irvington Publishers, 1986.

Cousins, Norman. *Anatomy of an Illness*. New York: W. W. Norton, 1979.

Critelli, J. and Neumann, K. "The Placebo: Conceptual Analysis of a Construct in Transition." *American Psychologist*, 39 (January 1984), pp. 32–39.

Derogatis, L. R.; Abeloff, M. D.; and Melisaratos, N. "Psychological Coping Mechanisms and Survival Time in Metastic Breast Cancer." *JAMA*, 242 (October 5, 1979), pp. 1504–8.

Dollinger, Malin et al. *Everyone's Guide to Cancer Therapy*. Kansas City: Somerville House, 1993.

Friends Can Be Good Medicine. Sacramento: California Department of Mental Health, 1981.

Goldberg, Jane, ed. *Psychotherapeutic Treatment of Cancer Patients*. New York: Free Press, 1981.

Goldman, D. et al. *Mind/Body Medicine*. New York: Consumer Report Books, 1993.

Green, Elmer and Green, Alyce. *Beyond Biofeedback*. New York: Delacorte, 1977.

Hall, Howard. "Hypnosis and the Immune System: A Review with Implications for Cancer and the Psychology of Healing." *American Journal of Clinical Hypnosis*, 25 (October 1982), pp. 92–103.

Holland, Jimmie. *Understanding the Cancer Patient*. New York: American Cancer Society, 1980.

Holland, J. and Rowland, J. D. *Psychoneuroimmunology*. New York: Oxford University Press, 1989.

Jaffe, Dennis. *Healing from Within*. New York: Simon & Schuster, 1986.

Janis, Irving L. "The Patient as Decision Maker," in *Handbook of Behavioral Medicine*, W. Doyle Gentry, ed. New York: Guilford Press, 1984.

LeShan, L. and Worthington, R. E. "Some Recurrent Life History Patterns Observed in Patients with Malignant Disease." *Journal of Nervous and Mental Diseases*, 124 (May 1954), pp. 460–65.

Leventhal, Howard; Zimmerman, Rick; and Gutmann, Mary. "Compliance: A Self-Regulation Perspective," in *Handbook of Behavioral Medicine*, W. Doyle Gentry, ed. New York: Guilford Press, 1984.

Liebeskind, John C. "Pain Can Kill." *Pain,* 44 (1991), pp. 3–4.

Locke, Steven E. "Stress, Adaptation and Immunity: Studies in Humans." *General Hospital Psychiatry*, 4 (April 1982), pp. 49–58.

Lynch, James J. *The Broken Heart*. New York: Basic Books, 1977.

Menninger, R. W. "Psychiatry 1976: Time for a Holistic Medicine." *Annals of Internal Medicine,* 84 (May 1976), p. 5.

Merton, Robert K. "The Self-Fulfilling Prophecy." *Antioch Review,* 8 (June 1948), pp. 193–210.

Morra, Marion E. *Sexual Side Effects of Cancer*. Bethesda: National Cancer Institute, 1986.

O'Regan, Brendan. "Positive Emotions: The Emerging Science of Feelings." *Institute of Noetic Sciences Newsletter*, 12 (Fall 1984), pp. 5–18.

Radner, Gilda. *It's Always Something.* New York: Simon & Schuster, 1989.

Roraback, Dick. "Cancer Is a Laughing Matter at This Clinic." *Los Angeles Times,* March 12, 1986, Section 5, p. 1.

Schmale, A. H. and Iker, H. "The Psychological Setting of Uterine Cervical Cancer." *Annals of the New York Academy of Sciences,* 125 (January 21, 1966), pp. 807–13.

Siegel, Bernard S. *Love, Medicine and Miracles.* New York: Harper & Row, 1986.

Simonton, O. Carl; Matthews-Simonton, Stephanie; and Creighton, James L. *Getting Well Again.* Los Angeles: J. P. Tarcher, 1978.

Sontag, Susan. *Illness as Metaphor.* New York: Vintage Books, 1977.

"Studies Show Hope Can Play a Role in a Patient's Risk, Illness and Death." *Medical World News,* June 11, 1984, pp. 101–2.

Temoshok, Lydia, et al. *The Type C Connection.* New York: Random House, 1993.

U.S. Department of Health and Human Services. "Management of Cancer Pain." AHCPR Publication No. 94-0592, 1993.

Videka, L. M. "Psychosocial Adaptations in a Medical Self-Help Group," in *Self-Help Groups for Coping with Crisis,* M. L. Lieberman, L. D. Borman, and Associates, eds. San Francisco: Jossey-Bass, 1979.

Walshe, Walter H. *Nature and Treatment of Cancer.* London: Taylor and Walton, 1846.

"Washington State Cancer Pain Initiative," leaflet published and distributed by the Washington Cancer Pain Institute.

Williams, Redford and Williams, Virginia. *Anger Kills.* New York: HarperCollins, 1993.

World Health Organization. "Cancer Pain Relief." Geneva: WHO, 1986.

Wortman, C. B. and Dunkel-Schetter, C. "Interpersonal Relationships and Cancer." *Journal of Social Issues,* 35 (Winter 1979), pp. 120–55.

Yalom, Irving. "Exploring Group Work Concepts: Similarities and Differences," in *Cancer and the Group Experience.* Los Angeles: American Cancer Society, 1976.

The Wellness Community–
National Board of Directors 1995

INDEX

Nolvadex (Tamoxifen), 221
Nutrition, and cancer, 172–74, 216–17
Nutrition Handbook, 213–33

Obesity, and cancer, 216
Objectivity, in examination of stress,
    39–40
Oncovin (Vincristine), 221
Organizations, 245–53
Orientation meetings, Wellness
    Community, 207–8

Pain
    control of, 125–31
    sexual relations and, 161–62
"Pain Can Kill" (Liebeskind), 126–27
"Pain Control in the Patient with
    Cancer" (Portnoy), 126
Pain Relief, How to Say No to Acute,
    Chronic, and Cancer Pain (Cowles),
    128
Pantothenic acid, 230
Participant Groups, 101, 104–5, 208
Participation in recovery, xvii, 4, 7
Partners, need for intimacy, 165
Partnership, patient-physician, 109–16
Patient Active concept, xvii, 8, 13–14,
    181, 197, 200–201
    physicians and, 182
Patient/Oncologist Statement, 114,
    210–12
Patients, viewed by physicians, 109
Patients Active, xv-xvi, 7, 14–15, 101,
    119
    and control of life, 67, 68
    and Directed Visualization, 47–48
    and quality of life, 19–22
    and reactions to stress, 41
    and secrets, 156
Personality, Type C, 143–45
Physical condition, and happiness, 21–22
Physical consequences of stress, 26
Physical treatment of pain, 128
Physical well-being
    emotions and, 6, 198, 200
    and relationships, 83

Physicians
    and pain control, 125, 127–28
    partnership with, 109–16
    and patient involvement, 181–83
    Patient/Oncologist Statement, 210–
        12
    and Wellness Community, 201–2
Placebo effect, 109–10, 117–20
    compliance and, 116
    optimistic expectations and, 146
Pleasant emotions
    analysis of, 33
    enhancement of, 50–57
    and immune system, 18, 27, 194
    See also Emotions; Stress
PNI (psychoneuroimmunology), 6,
    193, 198
    and Patient Active concept, 14
Portnoy, R. K. ("Pain Control in the
    Patient with Cancer"), 126
Potential partners, cancer patients and,
    164–65
Prednisone, 220
Prevention of cancer
    foods and, 173, 215
    psychoneuroimmunology and, 199
Problems, nutritional, during
    treatment, 227–29
Professional Advisory Board, Wellness
    Community, ix-x, 3, 181, 182
Protective foods, 224
Protein, 173, 215
    sources of, 224, 231
Psychological preparation for surgery,
    121–24
Psychological state, and immune
    system, 13
Psychological treatment of pain, 128–
    29
Psychology, Patient Active concept
    and, 14
Psychoneuroimmunology (PNI), 6, 14,
    193, 198
Psycho-oncology, 199, 202
"Psychosocial Adaptations in a Medical
    Self-Help Group" (Videka), 88